HOW TO CURE A MIGRAINE WITH FOOD

Morgan De Laurentis

Copyright © 2022 by Morgan De Laurentis

All rights reserved.

No portion of this book may be reproduced in any form without written permission from the publisher or author, except as permitted by U.S. copyright law.

Contents

1.	Introduction	1
2.	Some tips	7
3.	The book's about	17

Chapter One

Introduction

Migraines are something I despise.

Honestly, I mean it. This isn't only because I despise having them. That is only the tip of the iceberg. I despise them in every way possible. In fact, I've had a deep-seated aversion to them for the most of my adult life.

It wasn't until I was an adult that I began to appreciate them. She had a lot of violent outbursts. And I couldn't make sense of it either. She'll be alright in the end. The next moment, she'd be preparing supper or doing laundry, her face pallid and her eyes squinting, as if she was trying to hide her pain from my brother and me. She was never one to whine, and she never placed her own wants ahead of those of the rest of us. " Regardless of how hard she tried to keep it a secret, I always knew. I was able to read her expressions as well as she was able to read my expressions. And I despised anything that may give her headaches, as she referred to them. I wanted to assist so much, but I knew deep down that I couldn't. Of everyone I knew, she was the most intelligent and well-versed on migraines. Because if this beast wasn't contained by her at all, I was doomed to fail as well. No matter how many times I wished, I would still fantasise about finding the solution and destroying it for good.

Even as a child, when I started experiencing migraines, I detested them even more. Nobody forgets their first encounter with the beast; I still remember mine vividly. I was eleven years old and my class was taking an overnight trip. It was a journey I'd waited a long time for, but I didn't get a chance to really appreciate it. Without witnessing my mother's migraines so many times, I would have believed I was going to die. On the bus trip home, there were other kids having a good time, while I sat in my seat, curled up in my seat, and wished they'd just be quiet so that I could cover my eyes from the sun's searing rays. As soon

HOW TO CURE A MIGRAINE WITH FOOD

as I arrived at home, I vomited till there was nothing left, then passed out. There was a start to my relationship with the beast. The battle that had been my mother's was now my own.

My encounters with the beast were sporadic at first. Even if they became more frequent as I grew older, I'd come to accept migraines as a fact of life by the time I was in my thirties. For as long as I lived, I'd have to worry about the beast lurking nearby, waiting for an opportunity to pounce. I had come to terms with the fact that this was my fate and had no intention of changing it.

Migraines are still a family issue, despite the fact that they are becoming less common. As it turns out, my wife has them, too. In the same way that my mother perseveres against the odds, she does the same for the sake of others. This means she knows what it's like to teach a room full of second graders with her head pounding, each tiny voice a cannonball crashing against her eardrum. For the second time in her life, she has experienced the agony of having headaches nearly every day for the whole first trimester of pregnancy, refusing to take even a single Tylenol. However, this type of battle wears you out. Watching my loved one go through it was difficult enough for me on my own.

Likewise, when my one-year-old daughter began experiencing bouts of violent vomiting, I wanted to believe it was due to some strange stomach ailment. However, I had my doubts. I've known the beast for a long time and am familiar with its numerous disguises. So it was no surprise when, at age five, she came up to me and said, "Daddy, my head aches." with tears in her eyes. Her ancestry had already predestined her fate. Although I wasn't expecting it so fast, I wasn't shocked that it arrived sooner than I had anticipated. The beast had no mercy, and I was well aware of this.

That being the case, you now have a better idea of why I despise migraine headaches. Choosing a profession in neurology, which treats brain illnesses, may have made sense to me, as I am now tasked with treating migraineurs, or those who suffer from them. At the beginning of my career, a part of me believed I'd be able to find a solution that would assist my family, myself (and my patients) get migraines under control and lead normal lives again. Books, journal articles, my professors and my patients were all sources of information for me when it came to understanding them. Despite my best efforts, a solution for migraines remained elusive, but I was content in the knowledge that I was giving my patients every treatment option possible. There were several instances where it wasn't a great answer. But I felt that was the best that modern

INTRODUCTION 3

medicine had to offer. A few years ago my mother came to a same realisation: the beast could not be slain, but handled.

What occurred next, on the other hand, was unforeseeable. All of a sudden, everything appeared to alter in the blink of an eye. My struggle with migraines was finally gone. And it just so occurred. To my amazement, I discovered something that has entirely revolutionised my own life, has absolutely transformed the lives of many others, and will completely transform your own. As a result of this finding, I will be able to keep the promise I made to myself all those years ago when I was a child: the vow I made then to slay the beast. Finally, I've discovered its vulnerability and the means by which I might take advantage of it. Also, I'm very excited to be able to share it with you all.

A Study of the Monster's Character

Let me tell you a story about one of my patients who suffers from migraines to get us started on this topic.

Margaret T.'s Case

An accountant in her late 30s, Margaret T. has a strict dress code and is always careful about what she wears. Normally, she wouldn't leave the home without her makeup on, let alone without brushing her hair. But this isn't a typical day. Her decision to visit the local hospital's emergency room has been on her mind for the last month, and she eventually drives herself there, only to endure five excruciating hours in the waiting room's harsh fluorescent lights before seeing a doctor for less than five minutes. To add insult to injury, she leaves in the exact condition she arrived in. A nurse provides her discharge papers with instructions to see a neurologist the next day before she leaves. When I arrive at my exam room the next day, she will hand me this document.

This looks like a headache to me.

Her response: "Yeah, and they're dreadful."

Let me know if you'd want to know more.

A persistent aching in my forehead occasionally causes me discomfort." My left temple and surrounding my left eye begin to hurt with this hammering agony."

Do you know how long they've been?"

About a month ago, they began.

4 HOW TO CURE A MIGRAINE WITH FOOD

Has this ever happened to you before?"

As far as headaches go, I've experienced a few in the past. Occasionally, I have sinus headaches. Also, when I'm under a lot of pressure, I'll get one. However, they are nothing compared to this.

In other words, what are you trying to say?

This is the worst and most frequent case of headaches I've ever encountered." In most cases, when I have a headache, I just pop an Advil or a Tylenol and it's gone for the day. But these appear impervious."

"Is there nothing?"

I've found that Excedrin does help, but I have to take it constantly.

Do you take it every day?

Each four-hour period.

For the last month, you've been doing it every four hours?

"I think so, too."

"Yikes! Other than the headaches, are you experiencing anything else? "Do you have a special sensitivity to loud noises or bright lights?"

"Oh, yes, I'll need to take a nap in a darkened room," I said. Anyone who speaks to me is a complete turn-off for me. I've also vomited a few times since I've been feeling ill."

A printout of Margaret's brain MRI was given to me by the ER, where she was clearly preparing herself for bad news.

It's a scenario that occurs frequently in my office, and the dialogue nearly always follows the same course. A visit from the beast may be scary, even for those who are used to the pain of migraines. First encounters with it are viewed as a guaranteed portent of doom for people who have never experienced it before. But when they hear that not only are they going to be OK, but that—with a little effort—this beast can be battled and slain, they are relieved and even jubilant.

In order to defeat the beast, we must first grasp its essence. There are many misunderstandings about migraines, both in the general population and in

INTRODUCTION 5

the medical community. My goal in this chapter is to provide an in-depth explanation of what a migraine actually is and isn't.

Is There a Point to This Suffering?

In order for someone to truly comprehend what it's like to have a migraine, they must experience it themselves firsthand. It's virtually tough to think that something isn't severely wrong in your mind when you get your first full-blown migraine. After all, isn't there a purpose to suffering? It is meant to alert you to the fact that something is amiss within your body, allowing you to take appropriate action to remedy the situation. Whenever your foot hurts after stepping on a nail, your brain is telling you to remove the object before it causes an infection or bleeds to death. As a result, a throbbing headache must imply the same thing. That place has had a tragic incident, no doubt. Perhaps a quickly growing brain tumour? Is it a tapeworm that feeds on the brain? Perhaps more than one brain aneurysm has burst.

Actually, that's not quite accurate. While those items (apart from the tapeworm) can and can produce severe headaches on rare instances, the most common reason isn't quite that bizarre. Having to reassure my patients that this particular episode of awful suffering occurred for no good cause places me as a doctor in a difficult position. When they felt agony, it wasn't because their minds were in turmoil. As a result, when people look at me warily and secretly question if I earned my medical degree through mail order, I entirely understand.

I still tell them that. Having a migraine does not always mean that you have a diseased brain. It's just a series of stereotypical physiological occurrences taking place inside of otherwise healthy brains, and nothing more. If you've ever had a violent, excruciating pain, you've probably experienced this mechanism. When activated, it's a "very unusual" yet "natural" physiological reaction that happens in response to particular triggers. I say it's just a masochistic quirk in our psyches.

It's a challenge to get people to buy into it. I've been there and done that.

The Little Masochistic Glitch

In order to understand migraines, it helps to think of them as a chain reaction in the brain, resulting in a wide range of symptoms, including numbness, tingling, visual problems (such as double vision), nausea and vomiting, dizziness, exhaustion, and headache. That a process in our body may be set in motion by

6   HOW TO CURE A MIGRAINE WITH FOOD

a specific trigger is something we're all familiar with because it occurs all the time in our bodies.

As an example, consider a fever. It is the ever-vigilant white blood cells' task to identify invaders inside the body that first recognise a bacterium when it infects us. The release of molecules that elevate our body temperature occurs as a result of this first identification.

Think about the instinct to swallow. An impulse is generated when food strikes the nerve endings at the back of our throat. An electrical signal from the brain's limbic system goes to the base of the brain, where it stimulates a series of muscular contractions that force food down the oesophagus.

Both of these reactions are ones that most of us would regard to be natural parts of our bodies. A wide range of symptoms can ensue after the threshold for triggering a migraine headache has been crossed and the migraine switch has been turned, including, most notably, a pounding headache.

Even while we still don't know every little nuance of the process, we've made great strides in the previous several years in figuring it out. Despite its complexity, it has the potential for a large deal of variety, which has caused a lot of misunderstanding.

The Prodrome is the first part of The Glitch

Prodrome is the first stage of the migraine process, which can begin anywhere from four to 48 hours before the acute pain begins. Prodromal symptoms aren't experienced by everyone, and those who do may only realise they have them in retrospect. It is the most prevalent sign of a migraine prodrome that one feels exhausted. The exhaustion might be excessive for some people, and many will feel an overwhelming want to sleep. Mood swings (irritability, despair, exhilaration) and food cravings, as well as dizziness, diarrhoea, and increased or reduced urine, have all been recorded as prodromal symptoms.

Chapter Two

Some tips

The Aura of the Glitch

Auras, which can be scary but are very transitory, are a warning sign that a migraine headache is on the way for many people. At the onset of migraine attacks, auras are a sure indicator that the beast has been awakened.

All kinds of auras exist. Nearly every possible sort of neurological disturbance has been described as a migraine aura in some way or another's research. Disruptions in vision are the most prevalent, followed by those in the senses (numbness or tingling in the arm or face, for example). However, a variety of symptoms, such as slurred speech, weakness in a limb, dizziness, and even quadriplegia, have been reported. A notable characteristic of these transitory abnormalities in brain function is that they normally resolve within twenty to forty-five minutes after their inception. The first time you perceive an aura might be unsettling. Many people fear about having a stroke, and doctors frequently misdiagnose them as having almost had one (i.e., a TIA, or mini-stroke).

This discovery was discovered in 1941 by K. S. Lashley, a bright psychophysiologist and migraineur, who found it simply by carefully observing and studying his own migraine aura. A scintillating scotoma—a progressively increasing blind area surrounded by crescent-shaped light scintillations—was all Lashley saw before his migraines began. It's safe to say that this is the most typical form of aura associated with a migraine headache. In the beginning, the blind spot is modest, but it grows in a predictable way until it covers a large portion of the field of vision. Lashley calculated that whatever was happening in his visual cortex to cause this particular event was spreading across the brain at a pace of two to three millimetres per minute using his understanding of how the visual system is structured in the brain and his observations of his own aura.

HOW TO CURE A MIGRAINE WITH FOOD

Aristides Leo, a PhD student at Harvard at the time, produced an intriguing finding that looked to be tied to Lashley's theory in 1944 as well. Using rabbits as subjects, Leo was conducting research in the field of brain electrophysiology. It turned out that he could cause an expanding wave of depressed brain activity to radiate outward from the point of stimulation by stimulating a rabbit's brain in any method — electrically, mechanically, chemically. Guess what he came up with while calculating the propagation speed of this wave? A speed of two to three mm per second. The pace that Lashley had estimated in connection to his own migraine aura. There has to be something fishy going on there.

Since then, Leo's experiment has been duplicated in a variety of species. The physiological reaction appears to be common in the animal kingdom for reasons that aren't fully understood, but we seem to be the only species that can be aroused without someone rummaging around in our brains. This wave of depressed brain activity may now be observed in real time during the aura phase of a migraine, as reported by both Lashley and Leo, and spreads at the same rate.

We now know that the symptoms of a migraine aura are caused by a wave of spreading depression in the brain. Most of the time, the problem originates in the area of the brain responsible for processing visual data. Migraine auras may manifest as flashing blobs or multicoloured fireworks displays, or as strangely deformed things. When this wave of expanding depression affects other sections of the brain, other neurologic symptoms will emerge. An example of an aura is a sensation of tingling and numbness on one side of the body when the wave originates in the area of the brain that receives sensory inputs from the skin. Weakness or difficulty speaking may be observed if the aura originates in the part of the brain that regulates movement. A migraine aura can cause symptoms in nearly any portion of the cerebral cortex due to the fact that this wave can influence any part of the brain.

Auras aren't experienced by everyone who suffers from migraines. Some people may have them on a regular basis, while others may only have them once in a while. At least in some migraine sufferers, this wave of sadness does not result in a subjective sensation of an aura, according to research. This discovery suggests that the onset of aura symptoms may be preceded by a certain threshold of depressed activity, according to the researchers. There is some debate as to whether this spreading despondency is common to all migraines, whether or not they are accompanied by aura symptoms or not.

SOME TIPS 9

We now have a better understanding of the bizarre signs that precede a migraine attack. The good news is that they aren't quite as frightening as you would expect. However, we still haven't discussed why migraines are so excruciatingly painful.

The Pain of the Glitch

The brain does not have any nerves, hence it cannot experience pain. Though a migraine causes you to feel as if your brain is hurting, you're not alone. That, however, is really a compelling ruse. Where does the pain originate from if that's the case?

The meninges, a network of connective tissue that covers the brain's surface, can detect pain, as researchers have discovered. Dilated blood arteries in this tissue were formerly considered to be the source of migraine discomfort. These conclusions were drawn from studies showing a brief increase in blood flow to the brain following the cessation of the depression wave, which was made possible by dilated blood vessels in the cerebral cortex. Therefore, it was reasonable to assume that the discomfort was caused by the dilation of the blood vessels. Although the vascular expansion has long since resolved, it is unlikely to be the major cause of migraine headache based on more recent data.

Migraine pain is thought to originate in the brain stem, which is located in the temporal lobe. The brain-spinal cord junction is formed by the brain stem, which is located at the brain's base. Pain signals are normally received by the brain stem. Meningeal nerve endings that detect pain convey signals to the brain stem, which in turn transmits them to other parts of the brain where they are registered as sensations of discomfort or discomfort. This is how a meningitis infection (i.e., a headache) occurs, for example. It's a strange quirk of migraines that the signal flows in the opposite direction from the brain stem to the meninges. Technically referred to as antidromic conduction, this reversal of normal nerve impulse direction is regarded to be a key early stage in the production of migraine headache.

At this point, the nerve tip releases a variety of substances (such as substance P, neurokinin A, and calcitonin gene-related peptide) as it travels to the meninges. Meningeal blood vessel dilatation, protein spilling from blood vessels into the meninges, and meningeal inflammation are all caused, in part, by these substances. The meninges' pain-sensing nerve terminals are activated as a result of the inflammation, and the signal is sent back to the brain stem.

10   HOW TO CURE A MIGRAINE WITH FOOD

Is that clear to you? As it turns out, it's the brain stem that starts the pain signal it finally gets back! To put it another way, this is a vicious, masochistic cycle! A vicious circle is set in motion, with the level of intensity increasing until it either burns out or something breaks it, like medicine or a good night's sleep.

Part Four of The Glitch: The Aftermath

Those who have experienced migraines know that once the agony is gone, life does not return to normal. After the chain of events that just occurred, the brain and body need some time to recover. The postdrome is the term used to describe this time of recuperation. Fatigue or a general feeling of "weakness" is the most commonly reported symptom, much like the prodrome. Some people may have "brain fog," or the impression that their thinking is clouded. Migraine sufferers may sometimes notice that the bristles of a comb feel like small needles raking over their skin after the headache has faded. After the pain has gone, these sensations might continue for up to a full day.

What's the point?

In a nutshell, what I've just explained is the migraine process as we now know it. There is a biological response to specific stimuli, just as there is with fever or swallowing. In contrast to a migraine, however, heat and swallowing both have an intended function. The body's attempt to kill invading microbes with heat results in a fever. Of course, swallowing sends food to our digestive system for digesting. Isn't a migraine something else? Weird processes like neural depression, antidromic conduction, and sterile inflammation occur for a reason. Nobody can say for sure, that much is certain. In chapter 4, we'll talk about my personal suspicions. First, let's speak about how we arrive at a migraine diagnosis.

Identifying the Symptoms

Neither a blood test nor an X-ray or an MRA scan can determine whether or not you are suffering from migraines. Migraine is still diagnosed the old-fashioned way, with a solid patient history, despite the improvements in contemporary medicine. It is up to you to describe your headaches to your doctor in order to get an accurate diagnosis. Blood tests and brain scans may be used to rule out other, less common causes of headaches during a headache examination. These tests, on their own, are unable to identify migraines.

What are the symptoms of migraines, and how do they differ from other types of headaches? An formal diagnosis of migraines can only be made if you've had at least five headaches that fulfil the International Headache Society's rigorous rules (Olesen and Lipton 1994).

The headache must endure for at least four hours before it qualifies as a migraine.

Two or more of the following four features must be present in the headache:

- a decision made by one individual (i.e., on one side of the head)

the sensation of being alive

ranging from moderate to severe

- made worse by physical exertion

There must be at least one of the following two symptoms accompanying the headache:

vomiting and/or nausea

- hypersensitivity to sound or light (phonophobia)

A migraine with all of these symptoms is said to be a classic case. One of the advantages of using this checklist is that if your headaches fulfil all of these requirements, you almost certainly have migraines. Migraine diagnosis is extremely difficult to make based on criteria that are so exact and rigorous. The concern, however, is that rigorous adherence to these criteria would also result in a major underdiagnosis of migraines. If only individuals who satisfied these criteria were labelled with migraine, I believe the majority of persons who suffer from migraine would be given a different diagnosis. With no right diagnosis, we cannot hope to give effective therapy. The Beast disguised as a sheep Because migraines arise in a variety of forms, rigorous diagnostic criteria overlook many instances. The migraine process is made up of a series of interrelated events, as we've already covered. Once a trigger is set, it's a sophisticated process with numerous moving pieces and a wide range of possible outcomes. The severity of a migraine attack might vary widely depending on the exact timing and sequence of these occurrences. So the migraine experience varies tremendously among people and even within a single person's history of migraines. When it comes to the aura phase alone, there is a nearly infinite number of possibilities. As previously stated, migraine auras can be caused by a wide range of neurological conditions. In the same way, each person's experience with migraine discomfort and symptoms will be different. A terrible, throbbing headache is what most people think of when the word "migraine" is mentioned. However, the intensity of a migraine's pain can vary greatly. Dizziness and light sensitivity may be severe in certain migraines, although the pain may be minor. In the next, the pain will be intense and the ancillary symptoms will be nonexistent. It is only when the migraine process unfolds as described by the official diagnostic criteria—blurred or distorted vision followed by a severe, throbbing, unilateral headache accompanied by nausea and vomiting—that it results in the prototypical migraine as described by the official diagnostic criteria. In addition to missing an opportunity to intervene successfully, failing to detect migraine in disguise frequently takes us down a blind path, resulting in the loss of time, money, and effort. Thousands of dollars in diagnostic testing for stroke may be spent if an isolated aura of transitory weakness or numbness occurs without a following headache. When dizziness and nausea are the major symptoms of a migraine, the search for inner ear disorders may be useless.. When a person experiences a daily, moderate-intensity headache, they are likely to worry for months or years about the possibility of a slowly developing brain tumour. Thus, it is not uncommon for a patient who has just experienced their first prototypical migraine to present with a long history of episodic symptoms such as dizziness, malaise, fatigue, tingling in the fingers and toes, and so on. The majority of the time, these symptoms have been overlooked or misdiagnosed. It's possible that there is a lengthy history of headaches that have been incorrectly labelled. Headaches Caused by "Sinus" or "Tension": Real or Fake? It's a good idea to settle in for a while if you pick up a headache medical textbook and look up "sinus headache" in the table of contents. Although the term "sinus headache" is widely used, there is no official diagnosis for it. You may be wondering how this is possible. The phrase "sinus headache" is said to have been originated by pharmaceutical companies that were selling drugs for sinus disorders. They promoted the idea that headaches caused by sinus congestion were "sinus headaches," and that treating them with "sinus" medication would help them make more sales. While this strategy has been successful in selling a lot of sinus medicine over the years, it hasn't helped a lot of people with their headache problems. In fact, it may have actually been detrimental. The reality is, if we dig a little deeper into what most people call "sinus" headaches, we'll find that virtually all of them are actually migraines, with estimates ranging from 90 to 95 percent (Tepper 2004; Schreiber et al. 2004). It's not hard to see why migraines and sinus issues are sometimes mistaken for each other. For starters, the region around the nose, which most people refer to as their "sinuses," is frequently affected by migraine headaches. Migraines can be blamed on sinusitis if the pain originates in the "sinuses." Second, sinus congestion and fluid drainage from the sinuses are both

SOME TIPS 13

possible with migraines, as they are with an allergic response or an infection. With discomfort in the sinus area and sinus congestion, the phrase "sinus headache" is easy to understand. Sinus discomfort is a real possibility when there are issues with the sinuses. It is possible to have a feeling of heaviness in the face and even discomfort or tenderness near the nose if you have a full-blown acute sinus infection caused by a virus or bacterium. Fever, chills, malaise, and nasal drainage are all common side effects of sinusitis, which is caused by an infection. The sinus area may also be tender to the touch. To put it another way, if you're experiencing sinus pain, the cause and diagnosis are usually obvious. Allergies, in addition to causing sinus infections and congestion, can also trigger migraine headaches, further complicating matters. In the throes of a sinus infection or allergy season, migraineurs are frequently hit with a wave of headaches. Overdiagnosis of "sinus headache" is common, but is it really a major deal? Innocent over-the-counter medication that someone doesn't really need is the worst that can happen, right? Is that really that bad? Possibly. First and foremost, when we suspect a headache is caused by our sinuses, we begin investigating the possibilities. Our search is doomed to fail since we're seeking in the wrong place. But in addition to wasting time, misdiagnosing a migraine as anything else means that we miss out on the opportunity to discover and treat the underlying cause. Sinus drugs, on the other hand, aren't so harmless after all, especially when used during a migraine attack. Many of the drugs used to treat a sinus infection, including decongestant antihistamine and other sinus-relief products in combination, have been known to cause rebound headaches, which can be quite debilitating. After using a medicine to relieve a headache too many times, it begins to produce headaches of its own, a vicious cycle for which the only answer is to stop taking the prescription altogether. These side effects are quite prevalent, and most of the time they are the result of prescription medications. The issue is one we'll explore in greater detail in Chapter 4. "Tension headache" is a term that is frequently used interchangeably with "sinus headache." Anxiety-free headaches that are neither severe nor debilitating may be referred to as this type of headache. Chronic "tension" in muscles of the neck and face (often attributed to stress) leads to headache, according to the theory presented in this article. Like sinus headaches, no clear biological explanation exists for why this contributes to headache. Muscular soreness and/or pain in the head and neck can occur as a result of muscle tension or strain. However, this form of muscular tension and discomfort is rarely referred to as a "headache" by the general public. Tension headaches are often misdiagnosed as migraines disguised as headaches. Similar to sinus headaches, this is the case. Migraines can cause soreness or tenderness in the muscles of the head and neck, in addition to the sinus congestion they are

14   HOW TO CURE A MIGRAINE WITH FOOD

known to cause. Additionally, pain and stiffness in these muscle groups are two of many causes that may cause a migraine. However, in the end, the migraine sequence in the brain is the true cause of the headache. Effective treatment also necessitates an accurate determination of the underlying cause.

Or Who's to Blame for All This? "On the other hand, no one else in my family does." This is one of the most typical answers I get from migraine sufferers after their diagnosis. A normal reaction, as well. Disease and sickness are often viewed as "something you catch" or "things you inherit" by the majority of people. When it comes to catching a cold or developing emphysema, for example, we know that our family history has little to do with it. On the other hand, we become concerned about our own risk when we learn of the illness of a close family member. A migraine is viewed by many people as a genetic trait that you inherit from your parents. From this vantage point, it's logical to assume that you won't ever have one if it doesn't run in your family. A complicated interplay between our genes and our environment is the root cause of most disease. A person's genetic makeup may play a role in how sensitive they are to a certain sickness, but their environment can also play a role in determining whether or not they are vulnerable. When it comes to migraines, there's no such thing. While our DNA certainly play a role, it is only a small piece of the puzzle. First-degree relatives who suffer from migraines are more likely to suffer from them themselves. On the other hand, just because you don't have any first-degree relatives who suffer from migraines doesn't indicate you won't. Everyone is at risk of developing migraines. In other words, it's a physiological response that anyone may activate at any time. What sets one individual apart from another is just how easy that reaction may be set off in the first place genetically. All other things being equal, having a significant family history of migraine makes it simpler for the migraine switch to be flicked inside your brain than it would be for someone without such a history. Not having a family history of migraine isn't the same thing as not having one, since various factors come into play. There are several reasons for this increase in broad public knowledge of migraines in recent decades. There has been a significant increase in the number of persons seeking medical assistance for headaches and receiving a "official" diagnosis of migraine as a result. Misdiagnosis of migraine is so widespread that many people who suffer from it never find out they have it. "Sinus headache" symptoms may not be related to the pollen count at all. Your uncle's TIAs or "mini-strokes" may be mistaken as migraine auras, which he's had all his life. Finally, we often know less about our ancestors than we think. Often, my patients don't discover that they have a family history of a certain medical condition or sickness until they've been struck down by it themselves. No one is exempt from suffering from migraines. However, there are a few unusual types of migraines with clear ancestry patterns. Most people have heard of familial hemiplegic migraine, an uncommon kind of migraine in which one side of the body is permanently paralysed during the migraine aura and then has a headache. In contrast to regular migraines, which are caused by mutations in numerous genes, this particular variety is the result of a single gene mutation. An kid of a migraine sufferer has a 50% probability of developing the condition themselves. However, this is the exception rather than the rule, and most families are fully aware of the issue. A migraine is nothing more than the result of a brain function that becomes engaged. All of us go through it on a regular basis, much as getting a fever or swallowing our food. Only the ease with which the migraine switch may be flicked separates those who suffer from frequent headaches from those who suffer from them infrequently, if at all. A significant family history of migraine is simply one of several elements that contribute to your success in reversing the disorder. Migraine and Its Aftereffects Migraines are more prevalent than you would have thought, as you've probably noticed by now. This is also true. In the past several years, there has been a steady rise in the number of people in the United States who suffer from migraines (Lipton et al. 2007). Approximately 30 to 40 million people in the United States have been diagnosed with migraines. By alone, that's an eye-popping figure, representing billions of dollars in missed production as well as countless hours of agony. It's possible that the real amount is significantly higher due to the factors outlined in this chapter. We've been waiting a long time for a breakthrough in this area.

Chapter Three

The book's about

The Dreadful Threshold is crossed

the accountant from the previous chapter, misses her six-week follow-up appointment after receiving a prescription for sumatriptan. I'm surprised to see her at my office again, two years after the first time she visited.

"Good morning, Ms. T. For how long have you been away? When did you last check in with me? Inquiry, please.

The first part of the year was going really well. I took the sumatriptan you gave me a few times after my initial visit, and it worked well. For a while, my migraines were gone."

After all these years, they're back!?"

"Yeah, that's an understatement." It has been a long time since they returned."

"How often do they show up these days?" was the question.

"Each one is unique. On some weeks, I'll have a migraine for three or four days. A week or two without one is not uncommon."

If so, how did you find out what causes them?

The answer is both yes and no. It used to be that coffee would set me off, but lately I've found that it actually helps. If you get migraines, you may want to avoid foods high in monosodium glutamate (MSG), which is a known cause. My last time eating BBQ potato chips without getting a headache was when I was ravenous and had nothing else in the house. It's funny; recently I've started having headaches when I try to sleep in on the weekends. On certain days, I

HOW TO CURE A MIGRAINE WITH FOOD

have a lot of them during my period, while other times, I don't have a single one. The majority of the time, though, they appear to be unrelated to anything and just happen."

In a state of peril

The worst part about migraines is their unpredictability, which makes them much more debilitating. In order to organise our lives around them, we would need to know in advance when and for how long they are going to strike. In many cases, the psychological toll of not knowing if you'll be unable to work for a few days or a few weeks at a time is the most damaging aspect of migraine.

That doesn't mean we don't make an effort to discover the answers. Almost everyone who suffers from migraines on a daily basis will go to great lengths to discover what causes them in the aim of gaining some control over their frequency and severity. However, this may be a very difficult procedure. A migraine diary might be a time-consuming endeavour, but it can also help you identify possible triggers. Even when you've got it all figured out, things always seem to shift. Almonds may be your foe one day and your saviour the next. It depends on how you approach them. Even worse, migraines begin to appear out of nowhere. But what good is it if you can't figure them out anyway?

So, what gives? After all, the connection between migraines and certain diets and lifestyle choices has been extensively documented. Keep a logbook, identify the triggers for each migraine, and avoid them like the plague if that's the case. It should be simple. Despite this, many migraine sufferers continue to suffer. How can this be?

It doesn't matter what you think.

To compound matters, many people believe that each migraine episode is brought on by a unique factor, which leads to the idea that what brings on my migraines may be completely different from what brings on yours—and vice versa. Many migraine sufferers wind up searching for that one item that causes each and every one of their headaches because of this misguided belief. They'll blame it on the MSG-laden Chinese takeout or the glass of red wine they sipped over dinner. But what about all the headaches that came for no apparent reason, with no apparent cause? After a couple glasses of alcohol the night before, how did they feel the next morning?

A migraine is almost never brought on by a single factor. However, when the migraine threshold is crossed and the migraine mechanism is activated, it is the

THE BOOK'S ABOUT 19

result of numerous variables. All of the elements that put you closer or further away from your migraine threshold define your risk level at any given time. The migraine mechanism kicks in when your risk level reaches that point. In order to avoid ever experiencing a migraine, we must avoid ever crossing that line.

If you can envision flying in a basket tied to helium-filled balloons, you'll get the idea of how this works. As you fill your balloon basket with more and more helium, you'll soar higher into the sky. In contrast, increasing the weight of your basket causes it to drop to a lower position (for the sake of this exercise, just imagine you have a supply of balloons and weights you can add as you fly). The height at which you're flying at any particular time is governed by:

You're being dragged up by a large number of little balloons, and

2. The amount of weight that is dragging you to the ground. 3.

Then image your basket exploding into a ball of flames when you reach your threshold altitude (figure 2a). That's something you should avoid doing.

Figure 2a: Visualize yourself in this floating basket. Your migraine threshold is shown by the dotted line. Depending on the quantity and size of the balloons and weights that are pushing you up and dragging you down, the height at which you're flying at any one time may be decided. Once you go across the boundary, the beast comes to life.

This imagined floating balloon is now linked to migraines, so let us see how it works. The current amount of migraine risk is represented by the altitude at which you're flying at any one time in this specific comparison. What determines how near you are to (or how distant you are from) getting a migraine is a combination of all of the different elements. When your migraine risk level surpasses the two-thousand-foot mark, your brain bursts in the same way.

In order to prevent our migraine risk level from ever crossing the threshold, we need to know what things raise and reduce it.

To get you closer to the threshold are the balloons.

We'll go through all the things that can make you more likely to get a migraine in this section. Balloons are used to lift up our imagined basket. The chance of getting a migraine goes up every time you blow up a balloon. The size of each balloon will indicate which products enhance your risk level more than others. There is a difference between little and large balloons when it comes to raising your danger level.

HOW TO CURE A MIGRAINE WITH FOOD

Factors that can't be changed.

We can't control everything that increases our chance of getting a migraine. When we're born, we're handed a certain set of circumstances, some of which are hereditary. Others are things that we can't control, such as the weather.

Biological

1. A Long and Prominent Lineage

If you have a first-degree relative who suffers from migraines, you are more likely to suffer from migraines as well. However, it is simply one factor among several, and many migraineurs have no family relatives who suffer from the condition. a large-sized balloon

2. Hormones

This one is aimed particularly for female readers. There has long been a correlation between migraines and the hormonal changes that take place shortly prior to and during menstruation. The term "menstrual migraines" refers to the fact that some women exclusively suffer from headaches during their menstrual cycle. Pregnancy's hormonal changes can also be a powerful trigger, especially in the early stages. In reality, I've treated a number of pregnant ladies who have suffered with migraines. The good news is that migraines tend to become better as the pregnancy progresses. Birth control pills have been linked to an increase in the frequency and severity of migraine attacks in certain women (as do postmenopausal women on hormone replacement therapy). A low-estrogen pill can help some women mitigate this impact, while others will need to find an alternative method of contraception (when possible). Size of balloon: big (women only)

Congestion in the sinuses

Because of the high incidence of migraines that come with sinus congestion (either due to seasonal allergic rhinitis or a sinus infection), many people mistake this ailment for a "sinus headache."

Medium-sized balloon

Environmental

1. Smells that are overpowering

THE BOOK'S ABOUT   21

Migraine attacks can be triggered by a wide range of sensations, but scents are the most dangerous. Organic solvents, perfumes, scented lotions and creams, and other synthetic compounds are the worst offenders when it comes to lingering odours. Medium to huge sized balloons

2. Sunlight

Bright sunshine, particularly if coming in from an oblique angle (i.e., through your side window in the automobile), is a highly effective trigger for some. Make sure you have a doctor's letter to provide to police officers if you're pulled over for driving with tinted side windows. Small to huge sized balloons

3. Barometric Pressure Changes

When a storm is on the horizon, many migraineurs experience excruciating pain in their heads. The reduction in barometric pressure is suggested to have a role in the onset of migraines. Inconclusive results from scientific studies imply that this is a valid claim, but further research is needed. Small to huge sized balloons

Changeable Aspects

When compared to the other variables, these are the balloons that can be manipulated.

Dietary

1. Alcohol

Alcohol is one of the most powerful stimulants. How much alcohol you consume can affect your migraine risk, and the degree by which it does so is different for everyone. Some people with migraines may get by with just one or two drinks. For others, a few drinks are all it takes to cross the line. But if you drink too much, you'll almost certainly have a migraine (hangover headaches are migraines). There is a perception that red wine is a powerful stimulant, but I believe this is mostly unwarranted. Migraine risk appears to be influenced by the amount of alcohol ingested, regardless of where it comes from. a large-sized balloon

Caffeine is a stimulant (Coffee, Tea, Sodas, etc.)

This one's a little hard. For many migraine sufferers, coffee is a lifesaver after the attack has begun. Excedrin "Migraine" (as well as ordinary Excedrin, which

22   HOW TO CURE A MIGRAINE WITH FOOD

is the same medicine) and other migraine treatments include caffeine. Isn't it strange that something that alleviates a migraine might also induce them? Honestly, if I told you we had the solution, I'd be lying, but I do have my theories about what it may be (more on this in chapter 4). Caffeine, on the other hand, can both alleviate migraine discomfort once it has started and increase your migraine risk before you even have one. In addition, the time of day the coffee is eaten might have an impact. There are some migraineurs who can drink a cup or two of coffee in the morning without issue, but they can't do so later in the day. Caffeine's effect is situational, which is why it's so confusing. Caffeine is a stimulant. Add another layer of complexity by going cold turkey on caffeine-containing beverages, which is known to cause headaches in certain people. Medium-sized balloon

3. Chocolate

This one is also a tad challenging. Migraine sufferers often report craving chocolate when they are already suffering from a migraine, making it difficult to determine if the food itself is the cause of the need. The headache may appear to have been brought on by the chocolate if you eat it before experiencing any discomfort. In other cases, however, there is adequate evidence that chocolate can increase the risk level. Small to moderate-sized balloons

Tocopherol Acetate

MSG is a taste enhancer that may be found in a wide variety of foods. In Chinese cooking, it's a typical component that's used to boost the flavour. In many places, the "no MSG" designation is now prominently displayed; if you can't find this information, it's worth asking for a meal without it. MSG is a common ingredient in processed meals as well. It's always a good idea to examine the ingredients on the label if you are purchasing something that is not in the produce or refrigerated department (such as a box or bag of food that can be stored in your cupboard for months on end). Glutamic acid, glutamate, yeast extract, sodium or calcium caseinate, or any "flavouring" (e.g. "natural flavour," "chicken flavour," "beef flavour," etc.) are frequent MSG aliases to check for on the ingredient list. Small to huge sized balloons

Meats that have been processed and preserved

Meat that may be purchased at the supermarket and eaten without first being cooked is, in general, a danger (salami, pepperoni, ham, jerky, bologna, hot dogs, etc.). A common suspect is nitrites, which appear on the ingredient list under the names "nitrites" or "nitrates" and are suspected to be the cause.

THE BOOK'S ABOUT   23

Smoked meats and other smoked meals can also increase your risk. Medium to huge sized balloons

6. Cheese

Aged cheeses, in general, are the main culprits. In general, if it's a hard cheese with a strong flavour, your risk score is likely to go up. Since softer cheeses are less likely to have been matured, they pose less of a risk. Small to medium-sized balloon

7. Milk

Those who are lactose intolerant may experience mild to moderate reactions to milk. Migraines are more likely to occur when a person's diet is poor in fat. Milk sugars, which are more prevalent in low-fat milk, are the most likely culprit in this case. Small to medium-sized balloon

8. Citrus

Citrus foods and liquids, such as grapefruits, oranges, and lemons, can increase migraine risk. Consuming them alone and on an empty stomach appears to be the most dangerous mode of consumption. the size of the balloon

9. Bananas

Bananas have been cited as a powerful stimulant by some. On the other hand, I've found that eating sweet fruits on an empty stomach gives me a headache. As one of the sweetest fruits, bananas typically bear the brunt of the apologies. People frequently eat bananas to fulfil their hunger since they are filling, easy on the stomach, and require no preparation (which migraineurs should not do). Small to medium-sized balloon

10. Onion with Fermented Vegetables.

Onion consumption, particularly raw consumption, might increase your chance of developing certain diseases. Sauerkraut and other fermented vegetables have a similar effect. Although the danger from pickled fruits and vegetables is much lower, it is possible. the size of the balloon

11. Nuts

Some people are allergic to nuts of all types, including almonds, walnuts, pistachios, Brazil nuts, and even peanuts.

Small to medium-sized balloon

12. Fresh Yeast Bread

Some people have a difficulty with freshly baked yeast-risen loaves. Examples include fresh sourdough, bagels, doughnuts, pizza crust, and soft pretzels. the size of the balloon

The use of sweeteners synthesised synthetically

The most prevalent artificial sweeteners in diet meals and beverages, aspartame (NutraSweet) and saccharin (Sweet'N Low), are the most strong triggers in this group. Sorbitol, sucralose and mannitol tend to elevate the danger level just mildly. Xylitol, however, appears to raise the risk level significantly. Small (aspartame and saccharin) and medium (aspartame and saccharin) (others)

Lifestyle

1. Stress

Because it's so easy to point the finger at, this one is the most commonly cited cause of an attack. Modern life is rife with stress, to say the least. Who among us can get through a day without experiencing some level of tension? When stress is regularly blamed, even when it may not be justified, this isn't unexpected. As a result, stress (either mental or physical) has been shown to have a major impact on migraine risk. In certain cases, emotional stress presents itself physically in the form of neck and shoulder tightness, which can lead to migraines.

Consuming large amounts of food and/or experiencing large fluctuations in blood sugar

Meal delaying or skipping is a prevalent cause. Almost everyone who suffers from migraines has been in this predicament at some point. High blood sugar, which causes acute hunger, is more than likely what puts you at greater risk. Migraine is sometimes disguised as "hunger headaches" in my patients who come in for treatment after experiencing their first migraine. If you have a hunger headache, don't eat anything sweet! And I'm not simply referring to sweets. Your headache will get worse rapidly if you eat a piece of fruit that is sweet (apple, banana, etc.) Many times before I recognised that the problem wasn't that I'd waited too long to eat, but rather the food I was consuming as a means of satiation. a large-sized balloon

Disruption of the Sleep-Wake Cycle

THE BOOK'S ABOUT   25

This is a large one, as well. Sleep/wake cycle disruptions might greatly raise your risk. Sleep deprivation is the most common cause of this, whether it's due to a night or two of sleeplessness, going out too late on a Friday night, moving to a different time zone, or caring for a newborn infant. But it's not simply a lack of sleep that might put you at risk; excessive sleep can do the same. Some people don't think it's worth it to sleep in on a Saturday morning. Balloons of medium to large dimensions

4. Dehydration

Another typical cause is dehydration, or a lack of total body fluids. In the summer, this is more common after a long day outside or after a lot of sweaty exercise. Because alcohol is a diuretic (which means it promotes water loss through the urine), this is one way it induces migraines in certain people. Make sure to drink enough of water if you plan on spending a long period of time outside in the sun. You should drink plenty of water, but you also need to replenish your mineral stores, especially if you're a "salty sweater" (you'll know if you are). Drinking a sports drink is an option, but be aware that the drinks contain a lot of sugar. Taking an electrolyte tablet (which can be purchased over the counter or online) or a sprinkle of kosher salt with your water is a better alternative. Medium-sized balloon

Excessive Workout

Some people are triggered by prolonged, intensive activity, while others aren't. High-level athletes who train really hard are more likely to experience this issue. A migraine forced former NFL running back Terrell Davis to miss time during Super Bowl XXXII. Small to huge sized balloons

6. Sex

Migraine sufferers are more likely to suffer from headaches during or soon following intercourse than other people. Avoid it at all costs if this is the case with you. I'm kidding, I'm kidding. Taking an aspirin or ibuprofen (400–800 mg) before a sexual encounter may help you avoid this predicament. Small to huge sized balloons

7. Frequently Taking Migraine Drugs.

While it may seem counterintuitive, each time you use an anti-headache medicine to alleviate the pain, you actually increase your risk of experiencing a migraine in the future (all other things being equal). Later in this chapter, we'll go into greater detail about this occurrence. a large-sized balloon

8. Medications

Other groups of prescription medicines, including those containing oestrogen, can boost the migraine risk. I always encourage addressing your choices with your doctor if you're on one of the following medications, even if stopping or switching isn't an option.

• Inhalers for asthma/bronchodilators (albuterol)

— Stimulants sold over-the-counter, which are essentially caffeine pills (NoDoz, Vivarin)

- Stimulants prescribed by doctors (methylphenidate, dextroamphetamine)

Medicines used to treat heart disease with nitrates/nitroglycerin

Male infertility treatment (sildenafil, vardenafil, tadalafil)

- Acne treatment (isotretinoin)

The following is a comprehensive listing of the most often prescribed medications that have been linked to an increased risk of migraine. However, it is conceivable that additional drugs that are not on this list might increase the risk of migraines. There are times when drug withdrawal (under the supervision of your doctor) can help identify if a medication is to blame for an increase in migraine frequency. Small to huge sized balloons.

9. Depression If you are suffering from clinical depression, you are more likely to suffer from chronic pain since the two are mutually reinforcing. An increase in the frequency of headaches is an obvious symptom of depression, whether caused by severe depressive illness or an emotional response to an incident in one's personal history (death, divorce, etc.). And if this isn't treated, it's nearly hard to get migraines under control. a large-sized balloon

Almost there yet? Isn't that a long one? As a result, migraines are surprisingly prevalent. Nothing in my life has ever been without stress, and I'm sure that's true for you as well. No one ever stays up late or sleeps in. No one ever drinks coffee or alcoholic beverages. No one ever consumes chocolate or citrus fruits.

However, as the saying goes, knowledge is power. Fortunately, millions of migraine patients have shared their wisdom with us. And with so many different triggers, it would be nearly difficult to work out all of this on your own. " It's not enough to know what increases your risk for migraines; you must also know what decreases it.

Keep You Away from the Threshold by Using Weights

Migraine prevention strategies will be discussed in this section. Our hypothetical basket is lowered by these weights. When you gain weight, your migraine risk decreases. We can control a few things like the balloons, and we can't control everything like that.

Factors that can't be changed.

Not everything that decreases our migraine risk is under our control, as was the case with the balloons.

Biological

1. A Generous Family Tree

If your family has a history of migraines, you may be more susceptible to them, but if your family has no history of migraines, you may be more protected. You'll need a lot more balloons to boost your risk level if you don't have a history of migraines in your family, as compared to someone who does. Weight: a significant amount

Changeable Aspects

You may add weight to your basket and reduce your chances of a migraine by doing these things.

Lifestyle

1. Maintaining a Regular Routine of Sleep

Consistency is a problem for migraine sufferers, especially when it comes to sleep and nutrition. Maintaining a regular sleep pattern may seem like a chore, but your brain will reward you. Medium-to-large size for weight

2. Having a regular mealtime routine

Consider the preceding element. Make sure your blood sugar levels are somewhat steady throughout the day in addition to maintaining a regular routine (i.e, consistent from one day to the next). Avoid missing or postponing meals is

28 HOW TO CURE A MIGRAINE WITH FOOD

one method to do this. In Chapter 5, we'll examine the most efficient strategy for reaching this goal. Medium-to-large size for weight

Stress management is the third step.

Rarely do I meet a patient who claims to have never experienced a headache before. When I do hear this, it's usually from someone who isn't prone to headaches and has a very laid-back personality—someone who doesn't allow life's inevitable ups and downs disrupt their serene demeanour. "It is not the facts and occurrences that disturb man, but the attitude he adopts of them," stated the great Greek philosopher Epictetus. Migraines can be controlled if you can find strategies to properly cope with the pressures in your life. People who don't suffer from headaches may easily do this. As for others, it's a lot of work to get there. Talk therapy, meditation, exercise, and hobbies are just a few of the many stress-reduction methods that might fill several volumes. If you find yourself unable to manage your stress, anxiety, and worry, don't be hesitant to seek professional assistance. It's an essential part of managing your headaches. Weight: a significant amount

4. Breastfeeding

While breastfeeding, most women with migraines may notice a considerable decrease in their headaches, or perhaps a complete cessation of them. To make up for the fact that migraines are generally at their worst during the first trimester of pregnancy! a tiny to medium-sized person

Dietary

1. Vitamin B2 (400mg daily), Magnesium (400mg daily), and Butterbur

Products that claim to be "natural" are available over the counter (easiest to find at health food stores or online). Migraine sufferers have heard of just about everything, but these three supplements have the most evidence to back them up (Holland et al. 2012). There are no serious side effects, and the risks are low. In the next part, we'll go into more detail about these issues. Weight: light

2. Avoiding Foods That Set Off An Attack of Inflammatory Responses

We can keep the dreaded migraine threshold at bay by avoiding triggers that increase our migraine risk. Finding your major food triggers can be done in a variety of ways. Alcohol (not in excess) is the most common food trigger for nearly everyone. As for the others, there are two approaches to assess their significance. Keeping a diet and migraine journal, which you can obtain at ww w.mymigrainemiracle.com, is the first step to taking control of your condition. When you get a migraine, write it down in your journal and then check your food log to see whether you've eaten any of the migraine-inducing items we described previously. Additionally, you may use the Trigger Tracker app on your iPhone or iPad to keep track of and identify your triggers. If you have the willpower, another option is to eliminate all of the probable food triggers we've covered and then gradually add them back in, one by one. Whatever method you choose, the end result will be the same: less headaches as you learn to avoid the foods that cause your headaches. For one reason, you may falsely identify a food item as a main trigger when your migraine was actually caused by something else (such as a lack of sleep, the fumes of a cleaning solution, etc.), which can lead to misdiagnosis. One of the most life-altering and effective dietary modifications will be discussed later. Small to big in weight

Pharmacological

Prescription Drugs for Migraine Prevention

Many medicines are given "off label" for migraine prophylaxis, however only four treatments have been clinically proven to reduce migraine frequency. I'll go into further detail about these treatments later in the chapter, in the section titled "Ending a Migraine Attack—Migraine Abortive Treatments.". a tiny to medium-sized person

Let's take a look at a few real-life examples to see how our hypothetical flying basket might perform now that we know all the many elements that influence your migraine risk.

Jane S.'s Case.

About two decades ago, when Jane S. was still in her early twenties, she first began to suffer from migraines. She has gone to several physicians and attempted numerous therapies throughout the years for them. They have both had migraines, and she has concluded that they are inevitable and there is nothing she can do about it. She suffers from migraines on a regular basis, requiring prescription medicine three times a week on average. Jane describes herself as a "worrier," and she has a hard time letting go of concerns she has at work or at home. As a result, she has trouble sleeping on a regular basis.

The presentation she was working on for work kept her up all night one night, so she spent the rest of the night thinking about how it would go the next day. Jane slept for three hours instead of the normal seven to eight hours she requires. She woke up the next day with a knot in her gut. She made an attempt to eat breakfast but was only able to manage a few sips of orange juice. She noticed a shimmering blind spot in her right eye as she made her way to work. The pain in her head and stomach were unbearable by the time she got at the office. Although the presentation didn't go as well as she'd anticipated, she knew she couldn't skip it and pulled herself together just long enough to get through it.

In the days and nights preceding Jane's big presentation, let's take a look at her migraine risk level. Figure 2b depicts Jane's fictitious flying basket at the time of the drawing (see below).

A typical day for Jane S. involves a high level of stress, frequent usage of migraine medicines, and a hereditary disposition. As a result, Jane spends most of her time in a state of near-migraine apprehension.

Her family history of migraines, regular use of migraine medicine, and near-constant stress and worry all contribute to the fact that she is never far from her threshold for migraines. Figure shows that she spends a large portion of her time flying dangerously near to it.

Let's see how Jane is doing now that she's had some orange juice after a bad night of sleep (figure 2c). Jane's near proximity to the threshold makes it easy for these two things to push her over the edge into full-blown migraine zone.

Adding a glass of OJ and a bad night's sleep to Jane S.'s daily routine is all it takes to send her over the edge and into a migraine.

Joe C.'s Case:

Fortunately for Joe C., that's not the case. A headache has never occurred to him in his whole life, which is unusual given that he is in his late 30s. He doesn't know anyone in his family who has them either. Joe is a really laid-back individual.. Even when things are going against him, he can let it go and go on. He's not concerned about anything. Joe spends the most of his time (again depicted by the shaded region in figure 2d) far below the migraine threshold due to his fortunate genetics and calm personality.

Figure 2d: Joe C. has decent genes and an even disposition, yet even on a typical day, he is far from his migraine threshold.

However, for Joe, one week in particular stood out. A noisy new set of neighbours moved in below him the next week. Late at night, their apartment's sound (including the bass from their eighteen-inch subwoofer) tends to peak. Joe, who usually gets a good night's sleep, has been sleeping just half as much as he generally does since they moved here.

More worrisome, Joe is finding work difficult for the first time in years. Because of the cutbacks at his workplace, he is now responsible for tasks that were previously handled by three other employees. In addition, he's been consuming three times as much coffee as normal in order to remain awake at work because of his sleep deprivation. Fortunately, it's Friday night, which means Joe can relax for the rest of the week. A pizza (sausage and pepperoni) and a couple of beers and a bag of nacho-flavored chips are all that he needs to eat after a long day at work. The following morning, he takes a nap. His head is throbbing when he wakes up at 11 a.m. Nothing like that has ever happened before. After that, it's two more acetaminophens. Nothing. In a panic, Joe gets in his car and drives to the hospital, believing that he has ruptured an aneurysm. Once he arrives at the hospital, a CT scan of his brain is the first order of business. The results of the scan are normal. In walks the ER doctor, who proclaims that Joe has just suffered his first migraine headache. Joe is relieved to hear this. Joe has a scepticism. "But doctor, neither I nor anybody in my family has migraines," he protests.

Despite this, Joe's doctor is correct in his diagnosis. An entirely unexpected and terrible sensation has just occurred for Joe: his very first migraine. For a better understanding of what transpired, go to figure 2e.

It's been two weeks since Joe C. had his first migraine because of a lack of sleep and stress in addition to a rise in caffeinated beverages, alcohol, MSG, and preserved meats.

To elevate Joe's risk of migraine to the threshold, he needed a near-perfect combination of circumstances. However, the point is that migraines can still hit at any time, even if there is no personal or family history of them. Joe's headaches have never been an issue for him because he spends most of his time outside of his threshold. If he can find a solution to the problem of the noisy downstairs neighbours!

The Myth of Only One Trigger

Although this is a common myth, a migraine is never induced by a single trigger, as seen by these cases. Many distinct variables work together to put you at greater risk of developing a migraine. However, it is understandable why the

32   HOW TO CURE A MIGRAINE WITH FOOD

concept of a single trigger may be so compelling. Let's take a look at Jane's instance again to see how this works.

Finally free of her latest migraine, Jane began to reflect on the experience and attempt to determine what had brought it on. It all started approximately 30 minutes after she had a sip of orange juice. In the past, she'd gotten migraines after drinking orange juice, so she's certain she's discovered the cause this time.

Orange juice had just a marginal effect on her migraine risk; it was only the final straw that tipped her over the edge. To be sure, Jane abstains from drinking orange juice because she is convinced this is the cause of her migraines. She does not consider the influence of stress, irregular sleep patterns, or her frequent use of migraine medicine. That glass of orange juice would have made no difference if it weren't for these extra components.

A look at these instances will show you how complicated migraine behaviour may be and how difficult it is to pinpoint the "cause" of a certain migraine. A common misconception among migraineurs is that just two or three things cause their headaches. As a result, they spend their time and energy attempting to avoid those items. In addition, most migraineurs will experience a large number of headaches for which they are unable to identify a trigger and conclude that many of their migraines occur for no apparent cause at all.

Every balloon and weight is significant to everyone, therefore understanding how your current degree of migraine risk is influenced by each of them is essential if you want to master the beast. As impossible as it may seem, recognising your strengths and weaknesses at any given moment is essential for making sound judgments. Since your risk level is already greater than usual, it may not be the greatest time to sip on that glass of wine with your dinner since you've had a stressful week or a bad night's sleep. When it comes to menstruation, it's best to avoid alcohol for at least two weeks after the period has stopped, unless you've been sleeping soundly.

Keep your migraine risk level low as a general rule for all sufferers. We need a lot of weight to keep our imagined basket from tipping over, and just a few balloons to keep it from soaring skywards. To keep your risk level at a safe distance from the threshold, I'll go into further detail about the most successful technique. Let's begin by discussing what you can do if you happen to cross it.

Anti-Migraine Abortive Methods

THE BOOK'S ABOUT   33

While lying in your bed, your head is throbbing and you know you need to take medication for your migraine because your curtains are drawn. However, what exactly are we talking about here? Having so many over-the-counter and prescription alternatives is both a boon and a curse. If you make the wrong decision, you might be in for a headache for several hours or even days. Other considerations to consider are the cost, side effects, brand name, or generic. In the throes of a full-blown migraine, multivariate analysis is the last thing you should do. Even when you're at your best, it might be a daunting prospect. To help you make an informed selection, I've compiled a list of the many migraine drugs now on the market.

Abortion Pills Sold Over-the-Counter as "Nonspecifics"

Numerous over-the-counter pain relievers are readily available, and some of these can be effective weapons in your battle with a headache. All over-the-counter drugs are referred to be "nonspecific" remedies since the mechanism by which they reduce pain is not specific to migraine headaches.

Prescription pain reliever, aspirin (Brands Include Ecotrin, Bayer, and Bufferin)

When it comes to relieving pain, aspirin—a nonsteroidal antiinflammatory medicine (NSAID)—is the most often prescribed prescription in the United States. It's effective and inexpensive. Just keep your hands off the baby supplies. Extra-strength aspirin (500 mg each) is the best option, although it may be difficult for individuals with sensitive stomachs to swallow. Bleeding and bruising are more likely with frequent usage.

Other non-steroidal anti-inflammatory drugs (Ibuprofen, Naproxen)

To treat pain and inflammation in the body, aspirin and ibuprofen (brands include Advil, Motrin, or Nuprin) work the same manner in the body. Aspirin and ibuprofen both have comparable effectiveness in reducing a migraine episode and side-effect profiles. Ibuprofen's normal effective dose is between 400 and 800 milligrammes (two to four over-the-counter-strength tablets) while naproxen's typical effective dose is between 220 and 440 mg (one to two over-the-counter-strength pills).

acetaminophen (Brand Name Tylenol)

Though inexpensive and commonly accessible, acetaminophen is ineffective in the treatment of migraines. As a result, those who give it a try generally

HOW TO CURE A MIGRAINE WITH FOOD

take higher doses in an attempt to feel better, which puts them at risk for liver damage.

Adjunctive treatment

Caffeine's contradictory impact on migraine has already been explored. While it has been shown to increase migraine risk and even cause an attack in some people, it has also been shown to be an effective treatment for migraine, especially when used in conjunction with other painkillers. Over-the-counter versions include Anacin, BC Powder, Bayer Extra Strength Back and Body Pain (Bayer AM), and Excedrin, Excedrin Migraine, Goody's, Pamprin Max, and Anacin Advanced Headache (Anacin Advanced Headache). The acetaminophen, in my opinion, is a waste of time and money, since it introduces the risk of side effects while offering little to no benefit. Because of this, I recommend utilising just aspirin and caffeine-based medicines for patients who respond well to combination therapy.

As a side note, the aspirin and caffeine combo may be made at home. An aspirin with cola or an aspirin with coffee has been shown to be an effective migraine cure by a number of migraine sufferers over the years. In order to avoid a surge in blood sugar and the other damaging effects sugar has on the body, I would prescribe a cup of coffee instead of a cola.

Medications for the sinuses

During a migraine, some migraineurs suffer discomfort or congestion in the sinus region (the area of the face next to the nose), as was detailed in the previous chapter. They seek medicine to relieve sinus congestion because they believe they have a false "sinus headache".

These drugs may not help with migraine therapy and may perhaps make it worse.

What's the Difference?

Standing at the pharmacy's pain-relief aisle may be a stressful experience. In addition to the numerous brand names, most pharmacies have their own generic substitutes for each drug. They're also frequently a great deal less expensive! So now what? No matter how much money you save, you'll get what you pay for.

However, the active component in both generic and brand versions is same. Aspirin is aspirin, no matter if it's called Ecotrin, Bufferin, or acetylsalicylic acid at the molecular level. In other areas, though, the pills may differ. They have an exterior covering of some type, which makes them simpler to swallow and less harsh on the stomach. Brand names are more common. When it comes to the rate of absorption, brand and generic formulations might differ. This impacts how quickly the active substance enters the circulation. This might be the difference between success and failure in some circumstances. So, my advice is to start with a well-known brand. The next time you visit the drugstore, see if the brand-name generic version works just as well for you. Generic may save you money in the long term if it performs as well as the name brand. Just return to the branded product if it doesn't work out for you.

Medications for Abortion on Prescription

There are a wide variety of prescription migraine medications available for those who find over-the-counter remedies insufficient. "triptan" medicines are included in this category, which is the most effective class of migraine preventatives ever created.

"Triptans" is a migraine medication.

Migraine patients marked the year 1991 with a new medication. Sumatriptan succinate (marketed under the trade name Imitrex) was approved for the first time that year as a treatment for the physiology of migraines. Sumatriptan constricts dilated blood vessels and reduces inflammation around them by binding to particular serotonin receptor subtypes on the blood vessel surface. Despite the fact that it is useless for most other forms of pain, migraine treatment is exceptional. Those receiving 100 milligrammes of oral sumatriptan were rid of headaches after two hours in randomised clinical trials, compared to roughly 20 percent of those taking a placebo tablet (Carpay et al. 2004; Sheftell et al. 2005).

The first time sumatriptan stopped a migraine in its tracks was a life-changing moment for many migraineurs, including my mother. It was a lifesaver. A self-administered injectable was first introduced, followed by a tablet version soon after. Other "triptan" drugs have been released in the years since then. Serotonin receptors on blood vessels in the brain are targeted by all of these derivatives of sumatriptan. Most of their distinctions come down to how quickly and how long they stay in the bloodstream once they are absorbed.

Fast-Acting Triptans with Outstanding Results (sumatriptan [100 mg], rizatriptan [10 mg], zolmitriptan [5 mg], eletriptan [40 mg], almotriptan [10 mg])

They are the fastest-acting and most effective of the family of triptans, at the dosages prescribed. In terms of possible negative consequences, they are also very similar. If you're on a budget, go for the one that's the most affordable on your policy (i.e., the one with the lowest copayment). On many insurance plans sumatriptan is the cheapest alternative because it is the only triptan with a generic formulation. While the brand name is frequently superior, in my opinion, the generic (sumatriptan) is just as effective (Imitrex).

Triptans with a Longer Half-Life (frovatriptan [2.5 mg], naratriptan [2.5 mg])

It takes longer for these two triptans to take effect and remain in the circulation. For this reason, they are usually kept for the most unusual situations. For the most part, their side effects are less severe since they take longer to reach peak blood levels. As a result, migraineurs who are particularly sensitive to the adverse effects of triptans may find that these medications are a good option.

Preventative medicine for menstrual migraines has also been approved by the FDA for Frovatriptan. Taken twice daily for five days beginning two days before the expected start of a woman's menstrual cycle, it is indicated for this usage alone. I've seen a lot of positive results from my patients utilising it this way, especially those ladies who only have headaches around their period.

NSAIDs and Triptans

Nonsteroidal antiinflammatory drugs (aspirin, ibuprofen, naproxen) may be added to a triptan if the first medication doesn't work or just provides short relief. There are no major pharmacological interactions between these two drugs, thus they can be used together without concern. Treximet, a single tablet containing sumatriptan and naproxen, has been demonstrated in clinical studies to be more effective than sumatriptan alone. Insurance coverage for Treximet varies, however sumatriptan and over-the-counter naproxen can be used to imitate this combination.

Negative Effects of Triptans

Triptans, like me, can have mild to severe side effects in addition to relieving migraine symptoms. There is a sense of "heaviness" and "tension" in the neck, shoulders, and jaw, and it can be difficult to express what it actually feels like. Most of these side effects subside quickly. When the medicine is at its greatest concentration in the bloodstream, the effects will be most prominent, and they will gradually go away afterward. These effects usually last between 20 and 45 minutes. On the bright side, these side effects tend to coincide with the commencement of headache relief, so some people learn to look forward to their arrival and appreciate it.

That these unpleasant triptan feelings are virtually definitely caused by triptans' actions on serotonin receptors on blood vessel surfaces should be mentioned is worth highlighting. It is the same method of action that causes the unpleasant sensations that some people experience in addition to the relief from migraines. In light of this information, it should come as no surprise that, in general, the most efficient triptans have a greater incidence of unpleasant feelings. Throwing the baby out with the bathwater is the only way to get rid of them.

The Heart and the Triptans

Given that they constrict blood arteries, some people are concerned that triptans might increase the risk of heart attack, stroke, or other "vascular events," as previously stated. Triptans and vascular events have yet to be proven to be linked, therefore this issue is only speculative at this time. Because of these risks, triptans are generally not indicated for anyone with a history of cardiovascular disease, a history of stroke, or unmanageable high blood pressure.

In order to avoid the Stomach,

Some migraine sufferers experience nausea and vomiting nearly every time they get a migraine. Medications taken by mouth may not be the best option in certain situations. There are several reasons why you should not swallow a $80 tablet. For one, you run the danger of vomiting it out of your body. A slower stomach and gastrointestinal transit may also impede the medicine's absorption into the circulation and cause nausea. People who are in this situation may necessitate a delivery method that does not travel via the stomach. Thankfully, there are other options. Injectable Sumatriptan, as previously noted, is still widely accessible. Using a "autoinjector," the drug is injected subcutaneously, where it is then absorbed directly into the circulatory system. Nasal spray formulations of sumatriptan and zolmitriptan are also available. Again, the medicine is absorbed through the nasal mucosa and into the circulation without the need for a stomach to be involved in the absorption.

Ergots, a Migraine-Specific Food

Even though ergotamine and dihydroergotamine aren't specifically intended for migraines like the triptans, they are considered migraine-specific medicines. In contrast to the triptans, ergots are efficient in alleviating migraine pain but ineffectual when it comes to other types of pain. Migraine sufferers may find them ineffective due to a number of circumstances. As a result, unlike the triptans, they interact with various chemical receptors, which can lead to a wide range of adverse effects, with nausea being the most prevalent one. A poor oral formulation choice since they aren't effectively absorbed orally. Self-administration might be difficult, although nasal spray, suppository, and injectable forms are available. In general, ergots are better to a triptan only in extremely unusual circumstances.

Opioids are a general term.

Oral opioids, which are all morphine derivatives, are pain relievers that work on all kinds of pain. Additionally, they're considered restricted drugs because of their potential for misuse and habituation. Some individuals may see an increase in their migraine symptoms as a result of taking these medications. In addition to their addiction potential, these drugs usually produce sleepiness, nausea and vomiting, and constipation, and for the majority of people, this means that they are unable to work or socialise for a significant period of time after they take them. Driving is also dangerous because of them. Aside from severe cases, they are of little help in treating migraines due to safer and more effective alternatives available both over-the-counter and through prescription.

Migraine Relief in a Simplified Manner

We've covered a lot of ground in this chapter, but this chart simplifies and simplifies the process of finding the right drug to treat a migraine.

A typical day for Jane S. involves a high level of stress, frequent use of migraine medications, and a genetic predisposition to migraines. Jane, on the other hand, spends most of her time in the shaded grey area, always on the verge of a migraine.

Since she has a strong family history of migraines as well as a near-constant state of stress and anxiety, her migraine threshold is never far away. Figure shows that she spends most of her time flying dangerously close to it, as shown by the grey shading.

Let's take a look at Jane's day after a bad night of sleep and an orange juice (figure 2c). This combination of factors easily pushes Jane over the threshold and into full-blown migraine territory because she lives so close to it.

THE BOOK'S ABOUT

As shown in Figure 2c, Jane S.'s threshold for migraines can be crossed with a simple glass of OJ and a bad night's sleep.

What Happened to Joe C.?

Joe C. is in a fortunate position. He is in his late thirties and has never had a headache in his life. He doesn't know anyone else in his family who has them, either. In general, Joe is a very laid-back person. When things don't go according to plan, he's able to let it all go. He has nothing to worry about. For the most part, Joe does not suffer from migraines because of his calm demeanour and favourable genetics (again, shown in figure 2d by the darkened area).

As can be seen in Figure 2d, Joe C. has an extremely low migraine threshold for someone of his genetics and demeanour.

For Joe, things took a turn for the worse during one particular week in particular. New neighbours moved in below him that week, and they're noisy. Around 2 a.m., the noise from their apartment, including the bass from their eighteen-inch subwoofer, peaks. While Joe is normally a sound sleeper, he has been sleeping less since they moved in.

Joe, for the first time in a long time, is experiencing stress at work. Having lost the jobs of three former coworkers, he now has to do the work that used to be shared among three people. Since his sleep deprivation is so severe, he has to drink three times as much coffee in order to keep himself awake at work. On the plus side, Joe has the weekend off because it's Friday night. For dinner, he eats pizza (sausage and pepperoni) with two beers and a bag of nacho-flavored chips because he is too exhausted to cook or go out. The next morning, he takes a long time to get up. In the morning, when he wakes up, his head feels like it's pounding. He's never had anything like it before. He begins with two acetaminophen and ends with four. Nothing. Joe gets in his car and drives to the hospital, convinced he's suffered a ruptured aneurysm. Upon arrival at the hospital, he is immediately taken for a brain CT scan. The results of the scan were normal. When the doctor from the emergency room enters the room, he announces that Joe has just had his first headache from a migraine. Joe has a scepticism. The patient protests, saying, "Doctor, I don't have migraines, and no one in my family does either."

Nonetheless, Joe's physician is correct. First-timer Joe had his first migraine, which he describes as "terrifying." As illustrated in figure 2e, we can see how this came about.

HOW TO CURE A MIGRAINE WITH FOOD

A combination of poor sleep, stress, and an increase in caffeine, alcohol, MSG, and preserved meats has pushed Joe C.'s balloons over the edge and resulted in Joe C.'s first migraine.

In order for Joe to reach the threshold of migraine risk, he had to have a near-perfect combination of circumstances. To reiterate, migraines can strike anyone at any time, regardless of family history or personal history of migraines. Because Joe spends most of his time outside his threshold, migraines have never been a significant issue for him... When it comes to those pesky downstairs neighbours, if he can find a solution

Deception that there is only one trigger

Although this is a common misconception, a migraine is never caused by a single trigger, as demonstrated by these examples. There are a number of factors that combine to raise your risk of migraine above the threshold. Despite this, it's easy to see how the concept of a single trigger could be so appealing. Using Jane's case as an example, let's look at it again.

After Jane had finally recovered from her last migraine, she began to reflect on what had caused it. She then remembered that it started about 30 minutes after she drank that little bit of orange juice. Now that she can recall a few other instances in which she had a migraine following the consumption of orange juice, she is certain that she has discovered the cause.

Although the orange juice was the final straw, it had the least effect on her migraine risk level of all the things she tried. Confident that this is it, Jane vows to abstain from orange juice, ignoring the impact of stress, erratic sleeping patterns, and a history of migraine medication use, which will keep Jane's risk level dangerously close to that for a future attack. That glass of orange juice would not have mattered if not for these additional factors.

As you can see from these examples, migraine "causes" aren't always clear-cut, and it's not always possible to pinpoint a specific trigger. As a result of the "single trigger" fallacy, most migraineurs come to believe that there are only two or three triggers for their migraines, which they then set about eliminating from their lives. Furthermore, most migraineurs will have a large number of migraines for which they are unable to identify a specific trigger and conclude that many of their migraines occur for no apparent reason.

Acknowledging how your migraine risk level is affected by each of the various balloon weights and balloon sizes is critical to mastering this dreaded headache condition. Knowing where you stand at any given moment can help you make better decisions than trying to avoid every possible trigger. A glass of wine with dinner may not be the best idea for someone who has recently been feeling particularly anxious or who slept poorly last night, since their risk level is already higher than normal. That glass of wine may not be too much for you if your period ended two weeks ago and you have been sleeping soundly since then.

In general, all migraine sufferers should strive to keep their risk of migraine at a minimum. We need a lot of weight to keep our imaginary basket from tipping over, and only a few balloons to keep it afloat. In the next section, I'll go over the most effective method for keeping your risk level far from the acceptable level. In the first place, let's talk about what to do if you do happen to cross it.

Anti-Migraine Efficacy: Migraine Abortive Therapy

So, you're hunched over in your bed, the curtains closed, your head pounding, and you know you need to take a migraine medication. What then? It's both a blessing and a curse that there are so many over-the-counter and prescription options available. Choose incorrectly and you could be in for a headache for several hours, if not days. Other factors to consider include cost, side effects, brand name, or generic name. In the throes of a full-blown migraine, multivariate analysis is the last thing on your mind. A daunting prospect even if you're at your most capable. In this section, I'll go over the various migraine medications on the market and make it easier for you to make a decision.

"Nonspecific" Abortive Medications Sold Over-the-Counter

Pain relief can be found in a wide variety of over-the-counter medications, some of which can be an effective tool in the fight against migraines. In contrast to prescription medications, over-the-counter medications are considered "nonspecific" treatments because the mechanism by which they alleviate pain is not specific to migraines.

acetaminophen (Brands Include Ecotrin, Bayer, and Bufferin)

A nonsteroidal antiinflammatory drug (NSAID), aspirin, has been a popular pain reliever for decades, and for good reason. It does the job, and it's a steal. There is no need to go snatching up baby supplies. People who are sensitive to aspirin's stinging effects should take two extra-strength aspirins (500 mg each). It's possible that frequent use will increase your risk of bleeding and bruising.

HOW TO CURE A MIGRAINE WITH FOOD

Other nonsteroidal anti-inflammatory drugs (Ibuprofen, Naproxen)

Both ibuprofen and naproxen (brands include Advil, Motrin, and Nuprin) relieve pain and inflammation in the same way as aspirin and are therefore similar to aspirin in both their effectiveness in relieving a migraine attack and their side-effect profiles. This is why they are so similar. Between 400 and 800 milligrammes of ibuprofen (two to four over the counter-strength pills) and between 220 and 440 milligrammes of naproxen (two to four over the counter-strength pills) is the typical effective dose for migraine relief (one to two over-the-counter-strength pills).

Acetaminophen (Tylenol) (Brand Name Tylenol)

Acetaminophen, despite its low cost and wide availability, is ineffective in the treatment of migraines. In their quest for relief, those who do try it often end up taking more than the recommended dose, putting their livers at risk of damage.

Adjunctive therapy

Caffeine's effects on migraine are paradoxical, as previously discussed. On the other hand, research shows that it can help prevent migraines and even cause them when taken alone or in combination with other pain relievers. Over-the-counter options include Anacin, BC Powder, Bayer Extra Strength Back and Body Pain (Bayer AM), and Bayer Extra Strength Back and Body Pain (Goody's), as well as Excedrin, Excedrin Migraine, Goody's, Pamprin Max (Anacin Advanced Headache), all of which contain aspirin alone. As far as I'm concerned, the acetaminophen is an unnecessary addition that introduces the risk of side effects while providing little to no benefit. As a result, those who respond well to combination therapy should use aspirin and caffeine-based preparations.

Remember that aspirin and caffeine can be mixed together at home without the help of a pharmacist! For many migraineurs, an aspirin and soda or an aspirin and a cup of coffee have proven to be effective migraine remedies. It would be best to go with coffee rather than cola in order to avoid blood sugar spikes and other sugar-related toxic effects that we'll discuss in more detail later on.

Medications for Sinusitis

As mentioned in the previous chapter, some migraineurs experience pain or congestion in their sinus region (the area of the face adjacent to the nose) when

THE BOOK'S ABOUT   43

they have a migraine. Those who suffer from the fictitious "sinus headache" seek relief from sinus congestion by taking medication for it.

Migraine sufferers should avoid these drugs, which do nothing to help the condition and may even make it worse.

What's the difference between a brand name and a generic?

A trip to the pharmacy's pain reliever section can be overwhelming. There are multiple brand names for each medication, but most pharmacies have their own generic substitutes. In addition, they are frequently much less expensive! So, what are we to do? What's the difference between getting a good deal and getting what you pay for?

However, the active ingredient in both generic and brand-name versions is exactly alike. There is no difference in the molecular structure of acetylsalicylic acid (Acetylsal) or Ecotrin (Ecotrin). In other areas, however, the pills may be different. This means that they are more likely to have a coating on the outside, which makes them easier to swallow and more gentle on the stomach. Additionally, the rate of absorption between brand and generic formulations can differ, which affects how quickly an active ingredient enters the bloodstream. The difference between success and failure may hinge on this. As a result, I'd suggest starting with a well-known brand. If you've found a medication that consistently helps you, you might want to consider purchasing the generic version from the pharmacy the next time around. This could save you a lot of money in the long run if generic works just as well. If it doesn't work out, you can always return to the branded product and only lose a few dollars in the process.

Prescription Drugs for Abortion

Migraine medications prescribed by a doctor are available for those who find over-the-counter treatments ineffective. "triptan" medications, the most effective migraine preventatives ever developed, are included in this group.

Triptans are a type of medication used to treat migraines.

For migraine sufferers, 1991 was a turning point. This year saw the release of the first migraine-specific drug, sumatriptan succinate (marketed under the brand name Imitrex). As a serotonin receptor subtype agonist, sumatriptan works by constricting dilated blood vessels and decreasing inflammation around them. Even though it isn't good for other types of pain, migraines benefit greatly from

44   HOW TO CURE A MIGRAINE WITH FOOD

its use. Study participants who took oral sumatriptan (100 milligrammes) were free of headaches within two hours, compared to only 20 percent of those who took placebos (Carpay et al. 2004; Sheftell et al. 2005).

Sumatriptan was the first migraine medication that ever aborted a full-blown migraine for many people, including my mother. That and it was a godsend.." Self-injecting injections were first introduced, followed by pills in the following months.. Six additional "triptan" medications have been introduced since then. They all work by binding to specific serotonin receptors on cranial blood vessels, just like the original sumatriptan. Differences in absorption and blood circulation time are the primary determinants of their effects.

Highly Effective Triptans That Act Quickly (sumatriptan [100 mg], rizatriptan [10 mg], zolmitriptan [5 mg], eletriptan [40 mg], almotriptan [10 mg])

Fastest-acting and most effective medication in the triptan family are these five triptans. They may also have similar negative consequences. It's best to go with the cheapest option available on your insurance plan (i.e., the one with the lowest copayment). Since sumatriptan has a generic formulation, it is the most affordable triptan on many insurance plans. Sumatriptan, the generic version of the brand-name drug, is often just as effective in my opinion (Imitrex).

There are more long-acting triptans (frovatriptan [2.5 mg], naratriptan [2.5 mg])

As a result, the effects of these two triptans are more gradual and their duration in the systemic circulation is greater. For this reason, they are usually reserved for the most unusual situations. Their adverse effects are usually less severe because they take longer to peak in the bloodstream. Since they have fewer side effects than triptans, they may be a good option for migraineurs who are particularly sensitive to them.

Additionally, Frovatriptan has been approved by the FDA for the treatment of menstrual migraines. Two days before the expected start of a woman's menstrual cycle, it is taken twice daily for five days for this purpose. The women who only get migraines during their menstrual cycle have had great success with this method.

NSAIDs in addition to triptans

People who are not consistently relieved by a triptan alone or who are only temporarily relieved by aspirin, ibuprofen, or naproxen may benefit from a triptan and nonsteroidal antiinflammatory (NSAID) medication. It is safe to take these two medications together because they have no significant drug interactions. Clinical trials have shown that the combination of sumatriptan and naproxen, marketed as Treximet, is more effective than sumatriptan alone. However, insurance coverage for Treximet varies, and you can replicate this combination on your own by using sumatriptan and naproxen over the counter.

Consequences of Taking Triptans

As well as providing relief from migraines, triptans can cause mild to moderate side effects in some people (like me). Pressure or tension in the neck, shoulders or jaw, or a "heaviness" in the body are common descriptions of the sensation. Fortunately, the side effects are usually only temporary. Also, the effects will diminish after the drug has reached its peak in the bloodstream, which is why they are dose-dependent. These side effects usually last for 20 to 45 minutes at a time on most people. On the bright side, these side effects tend to coincide with the onset of headache relief, so some people learn to look forward to their appearance.

Triptans' effects on serotonin receptors on the surface of blood vessels most likely cause these particular unpleasant triptan sensations. It is the same mechanism of action that causes the unpleasant sensations that some people experience as a result of the migraine relief. As a result, it should come as no surprise that the most effective triptans are also associated with a higher incidence of temporary unpleasant sensations. These would necessitate throwing the baby out with the bathwater in order to get rid of them.

Tranquillity and the Throat

Given that they constrict blood vessels, some people worry that triptans could increase the risk of heart attack, stroke, or other "vascular events," as previously mentioned. At this point in time, this is only a theoretical concern, as there is no evidence that triptans are linked to vascular events. Because of these concerns, triptans are not typically recommended for those with a history of heart disease, stroke or uncontrolled high blood pressure.

Stomach evasion

Nausea and vomiting are almost always present in migraines for some people. Orally administered drugs may not be the best choice in certain circumstances. For starters, if you vomit the pill out of your stomach, you'll be left with a $80 pill floating about in your toilet bowl. It is also possible that nausea is a sign of decreased absorption of the medication because of sluggish digestion and gastrointestinal transit. As a result, persons in this situation may necessitate a method of delivery that avoids the stomach. The good news is that these other options exist. Sumatriptan, as previously indicated, is available in an injectable form and has been for many years. The medicine is administered subcutaneously via a "autoinjector," which allows it to be absorbed straight into the bloodstream. Nasal sprays are available for both sumatriptan and zolmitriptan. The medicine is absorbed over the nasal mucosa and into the circulation, again omitting the stomach from the absorption process.

Specially Designed for Migraine Patients: Ergots

There are two ergots that are regarded migraine-specific medications: ergotamine and dihydroergotamine. There are some benefits to taking ergots, but they don't work as well as the triptans in reducing pain from other causes. For the vast majority of migraine sufferers, they are ineffective. For one thing, unlike the triptans, they interact with several chemical receptors, generating the possibility for a multitude of adverse effects, with nausea being the most prevalent. As a result, the oral formulation is a poor choice since they are not well-absorbed. Self-administering nasal spray, suppository, and injectable versions are available, however this might be difficult. In general, ergots are better to a triptan only in extremely unusual circumstances.

Opioids are a general term.

Oral opioids, all of which are derived from morphine, are pain medications that work on a generalised level. As a result of their potential for misuse and habituation, they are also regulated drugs. They are less effective in relieving migraine discomfort than migraine-specific medications, and in many people they may exacerbate it. Sedation, nausea, and vomiting, as well as constipation, are all typical side effects of these drugs, which means that they can be dangerous if misused. They also prevent most people from going to work or social functions for many hours. They are very dangerous to drive on. Because there are safer and more effective alternatives available over-the-counter and by prescription, they are of little value in the treatment of migraine unless in the most serious cases.

Migraine Relief Using a Minimalist Approach

What we've learned in this chapter is summarised in an easy-to-follow procedure in this chart for selecting the best drug to relieve a migraine.

The "Miracle."

THE BOOK'S ABOUT   47

I believed I understood everything there was to know about migraines until the spring of 2010. Migraines had been a part of my life since I was a youngster, when I witnessed my mother's struggle with them and learned about their prevalence. In addition, I had my own personal experiences and those of my patients to draw on, as well as the numerous hours I spent reading neurology textbooks and periodicals. I used what I'd learned about migraines to help myself and my patients.

I felt confident in my ability to control my own migraines because of the wealth of information I had amassed over the years. Every single one of my migraine-inducing triggers was well-understood, and I had narrowed them down to a select few. One of the most prevalent was alcohol. Only seldom did I accompany my meals with a glass of wine or beer, despite the fact that I much loved the experience. The only way to avoid a full-blown migraine the next morning was to take a couple ibuprofen to ease the pain. But this only cut my chances of getting a migraine in half. For the most part, I had given up smoked or processed meats of any type, including sausages, pepperoni, and salami. MSG was also out of the question, which was a gift in disguise because it meant nearly total avoidance of the snack food section at the grocery store. I was only able to consume a limited amount of almonds at a time. In the morning, a cup of coffee was good, but not after midday. The lack of sleep almost always resulted in a headache, but I couldn't prevent it because I was on call at the hospital every fourth night. The one thing that always got under my skin was the inconsistency of my eating schedule. My schedule as a doctor is mostly determined by how many patients show up for their appointments and if I am on hospital call that day. On some days, I'd have time to have lunch, but on others, the mornings dragged on into the afternoons without a break. While keeping a supply of protein bars on hand was helpful, it wasn't always enough. When I was driving home from work, my head was throbbing.

There were approximately ten days a month when I needed to take a triptan to deal with a headache. Fortunately, I had a high success rate with abortive medicine, but it came at a cost. When I take a triptan, I may expect a few hours of tremendous exhaustion, which can make it difficult to visit patients or carry out my duties as a husband and parent. But it was worth it because the respite from the migraine allowed me to continue working, which would have been impossible otherwise. To date, I've only missed one half-day of work in the ten years since I from medical school. At the time, I felt that was a very decent result, given what I understood about migraines.

48   HOW TO CURE A MIGRAINE WITH FOOD

That was my current location. This migraine condition was the best I could expect for, therefore I was content with it.

In the fall of 2009, while surfing the Internet, I stumbled across a blog by Kurt Harris, a physician. It was a nutrition blog written by a neuroradiologist, which was unusual enough (a doctor who specialises in reading imaging studies of the brain). That was fascinating in and of itself. It was, however, the central idea of the site that truly drew me in. A low-fat, low-cholesterol, high-carbohydrate diet is not the greatest diet for maximum health, according to Dr. Harris. I'd been preaching to my patients for a decade about the dangers of a low-carbohydrate, high-fat diet, and I'd come to believe that it was the root cause of many of the diseases that we see the most frequently in our practise. Harris promoted a food and nutrition strategy that I would have regarded as blatantly ludicrous if it had been presented by anybody other than Harris. No matter how hard I looked, I couldn't find any grounds to reject it. Despite the fact that it contradicted much of what I had been taught in medical school, it made perfect sense. I came to the conclusion that I owed it to my patients and myself to go a bit further.

To begin, doctors-in-training receive very little official instruction on food and nutrition, which may come as a shock to some. In medical school, these are viewed as a waste of time, as if they weren't relevant to our careers as doctors, and as if they could be learned in a single lecture or two. We were taught that there are two important principles to keep in mind during our training.

One of these was that a diet low in fat and cholesterol is the greatest way to avoid vascular disease, which is the direct cause of heart attack and stroke.

Overeating and being lazy are two more contributing factors to obesity, according to this theory. You will gain weight if your daily caloric intake exceeds your daily caloric expenditure.

Our patients should eat low-fat meals and control their calorie intake, according to this directive. Done. The next topic is. Something as crucial to our well-being as the food we eat every day should be given more consideration. Because most physicians see it as an unnecessary distraction from more serious issues, such as damaged blood vessels, they tend to overlook it.

It dawned on me after reading Dr. Harris' blog that the nutritional advice I was giving patients was based on an unreliable basis. As most physicians, I hadn't done the necessary investigation to independently verify the material

THE BOOK'S ABOUT 49

for myself like most doctors do. For something so important to the health of my patients, this was an unforgivable omission.

So, with my eyes wide open and my curiosity piqued, I made the decision to delve headfirst into the world of nutrition. It was a must-read for medical students and one I suggest to everyone interested in human health and nutrition that I started with Gary Taubes' Good Calories, Bad Calories (2007). To better understand the epidemiological data on the relationship between fat, cholesterol, and heart disease, I re-read the book, which prompted me to go into biochemistry and endocrinology's finer aspects as well as human anthropology and evolutionary biology's novel viewpoints. I'll read anything that will provide light on what we, as a species, should be eating. In an area plagued by shoddy research papers and shoddy findings, I was determined to uncover the truth.

I prefer to have an open mind and evaluate all sides before deciding on a course of action. However, I felt troubled when I emerged from this activity. It bothered me that what I'd learned in school was so different from what actually happened in the real world. I couldn't believe how far I'd gone astray in my conception of what constitutes a balanced diet. I couldn't shake the feeling that I'd been leading my patients astray unintentionally all this time. Until recently, I was offering patients nutritional advice that was unquestionably harming their health and unknowingly feeding the same diseases we are attempting to treat, along with the rest of the mainstream medical establishment.

I made a decision based on the fresh facts I had acquired. As a result, in the spring of 2010 I began a complete overhaul of my diet. Not for the purpose of losing weight. I didn't do it to "feel better." I did it because I wanted to. I decided to do so after a thorough assessment of the scientific literature, which convinced me that it was the best course of action for long-term health and well-being. It would give me the best shot for a long and happy life.

As it turned out, I started to feel better after making this modification. In fact, it's far better. Having more energy was the first change I noticed. My erratic energy levels, which I had accepted as an inescapable part of life, were long gone. For as long as I can remember, I've always struggled to get through the afternoons at work since I was always so drowsy after lunch. I'm not going to say it anymore. In addition, I realised that my stomach no longer felt bloated after I'd eaten. The indigestion I had considered a normal consequence of eating a big meal was gone. My "spare tyre" around my waist, which had been steadily accumulating since high school, began to vanish after a few weeks. My waist

HOW TO CURE A MIGRAINE WITH FOOD

size was one size lower than it was in my senior year of high school when the fat reduction eventually levelled off.

It was a surprise to me, and I had no intention of losing weight or improving my health. I was simply following a diet that I had read about and believed to be the best for my overall well-being. In any event, these advantages were a wonderful surprise. But after a few weeks of following this new diet, I began to notice something else...

I hadn't had a headache. Neither a mild nor a moderate one. Though interesting, I remained sceptical, believing that it was most likely an accident. There must be a better way to get rid of migraines than this. After all, I should be able to tell whether it was. For crying out loud, I was an authority on the topic!

Then two months passed by. There was no pain in my head. Three months have passed since the last update. On to number four, five, and six...

The beast vanished in an instant.

Many of the stimuli that would have caused a headache in the past no longer did so, making my migraines disappear. Drinking wine with supper has become my new ritual. I was able to have a nut-based snack again. Sausage or charcuterie would be ok with me. Having a cup of coffee in the morning and afternoon would be OK with me. I no longer had a pounding head because of the lifestyle considerations I stated previously. An exhausting night's sleep no longer required a triptan to get through the next day. In addition, my inconsistent mealtimes, which were the most common trigger for me, were no longer an issue. Incredibly, I was able to endure lengthy amounts of time without hunger pangs and without the slightest hint of a headache.

Between fifty and sixty times a year, I would take prescription migraine medicine. Only once did I use it in the year after that, and it was while dining out (when I "cheated").

Putting into words how transformative this experience has been is impossible. In fact, if I hadn't experienced it myself, I never would have thought it was possible. I didn't anticipate any of this to happen as a result of my new diet. There's no way I'll go back to eating any other manner now that it's happened.

Isn't it the best? You are not exempt from this fate.

You're probably wondering at this point what it was that prompted me to rethink my whole approach to food and nutrition. For some reason, I'm begin-

THE BOOK'S ABOUT   51

ning to suspect that the medical establishment has been dispensing damaging nutritional recommendations for the better part of the last half century. Let's begin from the beginning of the process to find an answer to that query.

Reflecting on the Previously Acquainted

For some of us, it's easy to forget just how long we've been on this world. Most of us can't picture living without the modern conveniences we've become accustomed to. Although our current way of life is relatively recent in the context of our species' history, it is still a very short time in the broad scheme of things compared to other ways of living. It is estimated that our first human ancestors emerged on our planet around 2.5 million years ago, based on archaeological evidence. Since then, their lives have been vastly different from ours. As was their food. Our pre-civilized ancestors were hunters and foragers who subsisted on the meat and plants they harvested from the wild. For our prehistoric predecessors, food was scarce, so they moved from place to place in search of it. They acquired their food via hunting and gathering.

Hunter-gatherers who flourished on this diet for two and a half million years passed on their DNA to the next generation. People who survived the attack were carrying their DNA. It was via this process that the human genome became finely tuned for survival in the diet of early hunter-gatherers. In contrast, the human DNA hasn't evolved much since those days, even if our surroundings have changed greatly. Our minds and bodies are still designed for best performance in a world that we no longer live in. '

It wasn't until roughly ten thousand years ago, a brief moment in human history, that our way of life began to change radically. Domesticating plants and animals at this period was the first step towards allowing people to cultivate huge amounts of food in a single location, eliminating the need to traverse the world in search of nourishment. For the first time, humans were able to remain in one spot for lengthy durations. We had the freedom to construct civilizations, to develop technology, and to produce some of the most beautiful poetry and music ever written. When seen in this light, it's easy to see how this new way of life became so popular. Our hunter-gatherer lifestyle fell away as a result.

Even while this change was largely regarded as an indicator of progress at the time, it did have some unexpected effects. The average height and weight of the population decreased dramatically (Hermanussen 2003). Our craniums shrank in size. Overall, people had shorter lives. Tooth decay, iron deficiency anaemia, and other indications of pervasive starvation are clearly seen in the skeletons of these individuals (Angel 1984; Cohen and Armelagos 1984; Molleson 1994).

52   HOW TO CURE A MIGRAINE WITH FOOD

As a result, we died sooner and were sicker while we were still living as a result of agriculture. You'd assume that the development of agriculture and pastoralism would have resulted in a healthier populace because of the stability of their food source and lifestyle. These findings, on the other hand, suggest the opposite. It's hard to believe.

A Strange Metabolic Terrain

In addition to ensuring a more reliable food supply, agriculture led to a significant shift in the kinds of foods that people ate. For over two million years, humans had been adjusting to a hunter-gatherer diet and internal metabolic environment that had altered dramatically. A food that we were not built for might have an unfavourable effect on our well-being, therefore.

Then then, we humans have proven ourselves to be a tough lot. Because, after all, we've lived on all four corners of this planet, we may be able to adjust to this new diet just well. Is there any way to tell if this shift in our dietary habits has had any impact on our health?

Hunter-gatherers of the modern era and the ills of civilisation

Even though cultivation and civilization had been the norm in much of the world by the mid-nineteenth and early twentieth centuries, certain isolated regions of the globe remained nomadic and hunter-gatherer. To see how people change their diet from hunter-gatherers into contemporary humans, we may go to the remnant tribes of humans who still live like our Stone Age predecessors. The end outcome isn't good.

The records of colonial and missionary physicians, many of whom spent lengthy periods of time providing medical treatment for primitive communities on the African continent, provide much of what we know about the health of these pre-agricultural populations. The health of these communities as they moved from a primitive hunter-gatherer lifestyle to a contemporary, Western way of life and a Western diet could be seen by these doctors in many instances.

The same thing happened over and over again. From West Africa's indigenous peoples to Inuit in Canada and Native Americans in the United States' Southwest, some illnesses were strikingly missing from every primitive community surveyed. Cancer was the illness whose absence drew the greatest notice. Medical missionaries, anthropologists, and explorers spent decades trying to find even one instance of the disease being present among the Inuit of Alaska, the Canadian Athapaskans in the north, and the natives of Labrador.

THE BOOK'S ABOUT   53

Unfortunately, they failed (Hutton 1925; Trowell and Burkitt 1981). To put it another way, cancer rates among Native Americans living in the southwest United States and northern Mexico were both astonishingly low — significantly lower than those currently found in the United States (Hrdlicka 1908).

Native Americans, on the other hand, lacked access to a wide range of medical conditions, including cancer. Diabetes, obesity, heart disease, stroke, asthma, stomach ulcers, appendicitis, arthritis, and gallstones were all conspicuously absent from the list of "garden variety" ailments (Trowell and Burkitt 1981). There were no illnesses that would pay for a cardiologist's Cape Cod vacation house.

It's possible that people in these prehistoric cultures simply didn't get sick because they didn't have access to modern medications and cleanliness. On the other hand, the average life expectancy of these prehistoric cultures was comparable to that of neighbouring civilised people, even if disease was widespread in both of them (Hrdlicka 1908; Levin 1910).

In addition, there was an unusual phenomenon that occurred when these indigenous communities began adopting a contemporary food and lifestyle. As a result of the shift, a wide range of ailments that were previously unaffected by the change began to emerge. These included diabetes and heart disease as well as cancer, stroke and obesity. Each time a group of people transitioned from hunting and gathering to a post-agricultural diet, they would be found together, pointing to the fact that they were all linked to one another by a common reason.

Over time, the idea of "diseases of civilisation" arose out of these discoveries. Civilized cultures only had considerable numbers of these illnesses, raising the question of whether there was something about human existence that was specifically responsible for their appearance. The one thing that remained consistent throughout all of these shifts was the food. Because of the agricultural revolution, which allowed humanity to establish civilizations in the first place, there had been a significant shift in food, and this change had caused unprecedented levels of illness among the civilised population.

For the first time, a French physician, Dr. Stanislas Tanchou, proposed that some illnesses are only seen in civilised societies after meticulously compiling data from death registers. According to Tanchou's findings, which were published in an 1843 paper in the medical journal Lancet and became known as "Tanchou's ideology," cancer rates rise in tandem with a country's "civilization" and its population. We should be concerned about the health repercussions of

54   HOW TO CURE A MIGRAINE WITH FOOD

our post-agricultural diet, as Tanchou's studies show. After adopting a contemporary diet, hunter-gatherer tribes began to decline in health and became more susceptible to disease. This is the most devastating indictment of our modern style of consuming food.

Much of this study on hunter-gatherer tribes and the concept of civilizational illnesses happened in the early twentieth century. For a long time, a lot of it was either disregarded or overlooked. In fact, it was never even mentioned to me during my four years of medical school. In the light of these findings' consequences for those of us who are charged with protecting the public's health, it's hard to accept that this is the case. If the medical community had been more informed about these results, our present mainstream diet might not have been so misguided.

One Hundred and Fifty Years Later

This argument may be reframed in a different way if we consider the narrative below. While out for a walk in the woods, you come across a honey badger who has suffered a broken leg. As it is, it's inoperable and unlikely to last long. And so, because you're a kind person and a lover of nature, you decide to take it home and take care of it.

When you reach home, you discover that you don't know what to feed it. Both of the following alternatives are available to you at this point:

As a first step, scavenge food from your fridge and pantry and place it in its cage, hoping for the best.

• Option 2: Do some study on the honey badger's native food and feed it that.

Which one do you think is the most logical?

Isn't the solution obvious? Natural diets are well-known, and we all know that each animal has a certain set of items on which it thrives. This is the case if we feed an animal its natural food. We know it will become sick if we give it food it hasn't accustomed to consuming. It's common for pet owners to keep a close eye on the food that their animals eat. When I was a child, I was scolded for feeding my aunt's dog some table scraps.

Despite this, we don't apply the same logic to our own dietary habits. Despite the fact that we have been consuming foods that are not part of our normal diet for the past 10,000 years, the majority of us have never considered the health

THE BOOK'S ABOUT   55

implications of what we have been doing. The things we take for granted when taking care of our dogs, we often overlook when taking care of ourselves.

Our bodies have adapted to a certain dietary environment, but modern agriculture has allowed us to leave that ecosystem and enter one that is new and unfamiliar to us. We're eating a diet that isn't what our ancestors ate, and it's making us sick. Hunter-gatherer cultures and illnesses of civilisation are clearly shown to be real by the overwhelming data on these topics. Astonishing that we were able to go so long without noticing something so obvious. Because of our predisposition to feel that we humans have a privileged position in the animal kingdom, we may have overlooked this fact. Alternatively, we may have forgotten how little time has elapsed since the Stone Age ended in human history. We can't expect to get better if we don't figure out what caused our illness in the first place.

So what is it in the modern diet that leads to disease? Obesity, diabetes, cancer, heart disease, autoimmune disease, and other diseases may all be traced back to what we consume. There are certain foods introduced by the agricultural revolution that we should investigate if we know that our post-agricultural diet causes sickness. Here are the people we should be looking for, should we?

Grains from a Breakfast Cereal

Cereal grains should be the first place to look for disease-causing foods in our modern diet, because the agricultural revolution could not have began without them. There would have been no pyramids in ancient Egypt if it weren't for cereal grains, particularly wheat. Beethoven's Fifth Symphony would not exist if it weren't for the grains. We owe our civilisation to grain, for better or worse.

Humans have domesticated these grasses of the monocot family so that their fruit seeds can be consumed. There are many different types of grains, but the most common are wheat, rye, barley, rice, and corn. In breads, pastas, cookies and cakes as well as pancakes and waffle-type breakfast cereals they are the primary ingredient. All of the foods that the majority of people consume on a daily basis were never consumed by our ancestors before civilisation (Cordain et al. 2005). Since the agricultural revolution, there has been a dramatic increase in the amount of grain consumed in the United States.

Why didn't our hunter-gatherer ancestors consume wheat back in the Stone Age? Because they didn't want to die, it's possible. Grains are poisonous and inedible non their natural state. Wheat and other cereal grains don't want to die or be eaten, in fact, as do most live things. Living organisms, like you and

56 HOW TO CURE A MIGRAINE WITH FOOD

me, have devised means of preventing other living things from devouring them in order to ensure that their genes will be passed down for generations to come. To get away from predators, animals use a variety of methods such as fleeing, scurrying, stinging, biting, and so on. As long as they are alive, they have the ability to protect themselves from being eaten, but after they die, they are typically vulnerable. When it comes to plants, they've had to come up with alternative ways to keep other living creatures away from them. It is the goal of the cereal grains to ill those who consume them.

Humans eventually realised that crushing grains into a paste and heating them up made them palatable. As a food supply that had been inaccessible for more than two million years could suddenly be eaten, this was certainly reason for considerable joy. Grass can be cultivated in enormous amounts on small plots of land, and it can be kept for a long time without rotting, making it an excellent source of energy and nutrition. Because they can feed a high number of people in an area that is relatively limited in size, they are an ideal crop for the development of civilization. Grain farming swiftly expanded around the globe, and it eventually became the foundation of the post-agricultural human dietary diet. Hunting for food is no longer an option.

But is making something edible the same as making it safe, or even "healthy?"

Displacement of nutrients is the first grain problem.

Most of the meats, vegetables, and fruits consumed by hunter-gatherers were nutrient-rich, whereas grains are nutrient-poor. They are a poor source of both micronutrients (vitamins and minerals that we need in our meals) and macronutrients (fats, carbs, and protein) (the carbohydrates, fats, and proteins that supply energy and support tissue structure).

Composition of Macronutrients

Carbohydrate, fat, and protein content in meals may be determined by dividing them into their component parts. Carbohydrates make up the bulk of grains. We may see that a piece of whole-wheat bread has 12 grammes of carbohydrate, 4 grammes of protein, and 1 gramme of fat, for example. Carbohydrates account for around 65 percent of the calories in a slice of whole-wheat bread. It is a low-protein and low-fat source of nutrition. As a result, we must eat foods other than grains if we are to acquire the protein and fat we need to live. Carbohydrate is the only one of the three macronutrients that we can survive without. Just protein and fat may keep you going for the rest of your life. Carbohydrate, or more particularly glucose, may be synthesised by

THE BOOK'S ABOUT   57

human systems from other sources. However, fat and protein do not fall within this category, as they are required for a healthy diet. As a result, grains are particularly deficient in the proteins and lipids that keep us alive.

Composition of the Micronutrients

All foods include a tiny amount of micronutrients, such as vitamins and minerals, in addition to protein, fat, and carbohydrate. Additionally, grains don't measure up when it comes to their nutritional levels. As a first step, they lack vitamin A and C, two nutrients vital to health and survival. Aside from the lack of B12 and the little levels of B vitamins (such as thiamine), riboflavin, and niacin), they also contain no vitamin B12. In impoverished nations, where grains are almost exclusively consumed out of need, devastating epidemics of micronutrient-deficiency syndromes such as pellagra and beriberi are not uncommon.

grains' relative lack of nutrients may pose an issue even in regions where people eat a wide variety of foods. To put it more succinctly, when we consume a lot of one item, we tend to consume less of another. So, if we're eating a lot of grains, as most people do these days, we're also consuming less of the nutrients our bodies require, such vitamins, minerals, proteins, and lipids. Supplements worth billions of dollars would not exist if grains weren't in the food supply.

As a result, many of us live in areas where nutrient-dense foods are readily available. Wheat is a poor provider of nutrients, but most meats, vegetables, and fruits are superior. When it comes to grains, there is no shortage of alternatives. The grains in our diet may, however, hinder us from fully reaping the benefits of a more nutrient-dense diet.

Antinutrients are the second grain problem.

Grains, like other living things, have created a number of defence mechanisms to prevent us from eating them, as was discussed before. These defences were decreased by current food processing procedures (or else we wouldn't have the ability to consume them). Grains, despite our best efforts, continue to put up a fight..

Bacteria and Gastrointestinal Perfection

When it comes to protecting plants against predators, lectins are the most common defensive mechanism. Plant lectins are still a mystery to us, but we do know that one of their primary tasks is to deter mammals from eating them. For

58 HOW TO CURE A MIGRAINE WITH FOOD

this purpose, they inflict on the animals who consume them a slew of severe side effects or even death. Grains and soy are among the most lectin-rich foods in the normal contemporary diet.

Let's use the lectin found in wheat, wheat germ agglutinin (WGA), as an example to better understand what occurs when we consume it. Other proteins it comes into touch with are quickly bound by WGA, as is the case with other lectins. WGA adheres to the intestinal villi once it enters our system (fingerlike projections along the walls of the gut that are critical for the absorption of nutrients). When WGA binds to the villi, it causes cell death and damage. Lipid absorption is hampered when lectins, such as WGA, destroy the villi in our intestines. Eating lectins has been shown to have a negative impact on the body's natural microflora. Our digestive system depends on beneficial microbes like E. coli and other pathogens that may overwhelm the natural microbial habitat in our gut and make us sick if they are disrupted.

Damage to the villi also disturbs another crucial function of our digestive system, preventing the absorption of nutrients. They aid in the absorption of nutrients, but they also operate as a barrier between our digestive tracts and other parts of our bodies. They are in charge of what goes in and what comes out of the body. A "leaky gut" is a result of lignin-induced degradation, which weakens this vital function. A leaky gut permits items that aren't meant to be in our system to get into our bloodstream. Before absorption, proteins are generally broken down into their component amino acids, however this does not happen. When our immune system identifies these proteins as foreign invaders, a cascade of events occurs that, among other things, causes the production of inflammatory molecules throughout the body in an effort to remove the invaders. One of civilization's most well-documented disorders, autoimmune sickness, is linked to the presence of these alien, undigested proteins in the body.

Phytates That Bind to Minerals

Phytic acid, or phytate, is the form in which the mineral phosphorus is kept inside plants, and it is abundant in grains. Phytate cannot be metabolised by humans since we lack the required enzyme. It also binds to other vital minerals, such as calcium, magnesium, iron, and zinc, on its way down our digestive systems. It is impossible to absorb these minerals after they have been bonded. It gets worse: Whole grains, which are supposed to be healthy, have the greatest concentration of phytates.

Autoimmunity and Foreign Proteins in Grains: The Third Challenge

THE BOOK'S ABOUT 59

When our immune system incorrectly attacks our own physiological tissues, it results in autoimmune diseases such as rheumatoid arthritis, multiple sclerosis, Crohn's disease, hypothyroidism, and type 1 diabetes. The immune system destroys joints in rheumatoid arthritis, producing severe inflammation and deformity. Patients with multiple sclerosis are subjected to attacks on the neurological system, which results in impairments in brain and spinal cord function.

Sadly, autoimmune diseases are becoming increasingly frequent. There's a good chance you know someone who has one, or you have one yourself. In addition, there is increasing evidence that many of these are caused by what we consume. Let us first discuss the nature of autoimmune disorders in order to better grasp how this occurs.

Our immune systems must decide which parts of our bodies need to be attacked and destroyed, and which parts may be left alone, in order to keep our bodies safe from invaders. The body is the most important thing to leave alone. As a result, there is a sophisticated mechanism in place to ensure that our immune system can tell the difference between friendly and hostile invaders. Mistakes will still happen, however. Antibody-mediated immune responses are the most common mechanism through which these errors occur.

Certain white blood cells in our immune system produce antibodies whenever they come into contact with a foreign protein for the first time. Antibodies may then attach to any foreign protein in the body and flag it for destruction and removal by other immune system cells after they have been created. There are many proteins on viruses and bacteria, and antibodies that specifically target these proteins are a main method for removing them from our systems.

However, a foreign protein may mimic a protein found in our own body in rare situations. Rheumatic fever is an immune system-mediated attack on the heart caused by an antibody developed to resist a protein on a strep bacteria that looks very similar to a protein in heart tissue. For example, microbes can cause an autoimmune disease even after the infection has been cleared up.

While viruses and bacteria include proteins that can cause the body to fight itself, it isn't the only one. Antibody-mediated mistaken identification and resulting autoimmune illness can also be caused by our diet's proteins, according to new research (Cordain 1999). Gluten is the most probable food protein to elicit this unwanted reaction.

60 HOW TO CURE A MIGRAINE WITH FOOD

Gliadin and glutelin, the two proteins that make up gluten, are found in wheat, barley, and rye. Bread's elasticity and stretchiness can be attributed to the presence of gluten. However, gluten can cause significant illness in certain people. Gluten intolerance affects an estimated 1% of the population, however most people are unaware of it. Celiac disease occurs when gluten-intolerant individuals ingest gluten grains. An antibody-mediated immune system attack on the intestines results in persistent diarrhoea, tiredness, stunted development, vitamin and mineral shortages, anaemia, neurological damage and osteoporosis in celiac disease, an autoimmune illness. More than only the intestines seem to be affected by the body's response to gluten in celiac disease patients' increased incidences of cancer, schizophrenia, and an array of autoimmune diseases (Jackson et al. 2012; Rubio-Tapia and Murray 2010). On the other hand, practically every chronic autoimmune condition we know of is linked to an increased chance of developing celiac disease (Cosnes et al. 2008; Rousset 2004; Rodrigo et al. 2011; Song and Choi 2004).

That being said, celiac disease is only a small part of the picture. The gluten intolerance of one percent of the population is believed to be a third of the population's risk of developing a mild form of celiac disease when they are exposed to gluten grains (Anderson 2012). The medical establishment is not aware of how widespread the problem of gluten intolerance is, and these gluten-sensitive patients may suffer for years, if not their whole lives, with a variety of inexplicable symptoms. That's enough to make anyone think twice about consuming gluten-containing meals. The gliadin protein in gluten may be the major cause of a variety of deadly autoimmune disorders, as well. In addition to curing celiac disease fully with a gluten-free diet (Kneepkens and von Blomberg 2012), anecdotal reports of people reversing other autoimmune conditions with a gluten-free diet are increasing.

Most, if not all, of us were never supposed to eat gluten, which was introduced into our diets during the agricultural revolution.

This is the fourth and last issue with grains: carbohydrate intakes and fat storage

Grains are mostly composed of carbohydrate, as previously stated. As long as we eat grains just sometimes, this might not be a concern. However, they are the principal source of energy for most individuals because of their role in the modern diet. Between 350 and 600 grammes of carbohydrates are consumed by the average American each day, most of which comes from grains. We rely on it as our major source of calories, according to the USDA food pyramid.

THE BOOK'S ABOUT 61

However, it is believed that our pre-agricultural ancestors ingested less than 100 grammes of carbohydrate per day on average due to the absence of grains and a few other current sources of carbohydrate. This is a startling rise.

What happens to our metabolism when we eat carbs? Let's focus on grains because they include a high amount of carbs. A vast chain of glucose molecules is what makes up the bulk of the carbohydrate in grains. Our saliva and pancreas release enzymes that swiftly break down starch into its separate glucose molecules. Absorption of the glucose into the blood causes an increase in "blood sugar."

In response to an increase in blood sugar, the pancreas releases insulin, an important hormone that aids the body's process of removing glucose from the bloodstream for storage. It is possible to burn glucose for energy once it has entered the tissues. However, even after the tissues have consumed all of the glucose, the blood still has to be flushed. Too much glucose can cause permanent harm to the body's tissues because of the way it adheres to them. So how does our body get rid of all this extra glucose? It stores it...in fat. That's correct, of course. If you eat more carbohydrate than you need, your body will store it as fat, thanks to insulin. insulin also restricts adipose tissue's release of fat as a result of its role in promoting the storage of glucose as fat.

So, contrary to popular belief, eating fat does not cause weight gain. The hormone insulin is responsible for storing fat in the body's fat tissues. It is glucose, not fat, that triggers the production of insulin in the body. In addition, grain is the principal source of glucose in today's diets.

In light of this, what do you suppose occurs when we contemporary, sedentary humans consume five to seven times as much carbohydrate than our hunter-gatherer forefathers, those same people who traversed the planet on foot in quest of food?

Greetings, epidemic of obesity. I'm glad to have met you.

As our carbohydrate consumption has skyrocketed in recent years, our insulin levels have likewise skyrocketed. Our bodies aren't simply accumulating more fat, but they have a tougher difficulty getting to that stored fat for energy because of the metabolic impacts of carbohydrate. So, despite the fact that fat cells store a lot of energy, a high-carbohydrate diet prevents you from accessing it. Energy requirements were mostly satisfied by fat burning in our ancestors' low-carbohydrate diets, which explains why they were not obese. Most of our stored fat is unable to be accessed in the current, grain-based,

62   HOW TO CURE A MIGRAINE WITH FOOD

high-carbohydrate diet. Instead, we must rely on the glucose in our next meal to power our bodies, and so the cycle goes.

Final Word on Grains

Now that the data is in, it's safe to say that grains are in the doghouse. Furthermore, they have obvious and logical methods by which they are linked to illnesses of civilization, making them a minor portion of the human diet before agriculture. Grains, particularly those heavy in gluten and phytates, are clearly not worthy of their current reputation as an essential element of a "healthy diet," given their lack of nutritional value.

Sugar is a likely suspect number two.

Sugar. heavenly sugar Almost everyone enjoys this. It enhances the flavour of our beverages and doughnuts. Of course, few would claim that sugar is genuinely beneficial. Neither protein nor fat are present in it. Carbohydrate is the only ingredient in this "empty calorie," which provides just a small amount of energy to the body. Sugar isn't a healthy diet staple, but it's not harmful in any other way. Right?

Humans didn't consume a lot of sugar prior to the agricultural revolution. Even while it wasn't that they didn't like food, our forefathers just didn't have the opportunity to eat as much as we do now. Fructose from the fruits they found or, for those who were lucky enough to dwell in the proper area, some wild honey were the two most common ways they consumed it. A year's worth of sugar consumption by modern people is estimated at two to four pounds, based on data from hunter-gatherer societies of the past.

It's a whole different world now. There's sugar all over the place. Sugar consumption in the United States has risen to an almost unimaginable level of 150 pounds or more per year per person (USDA 2003). Over our hunter-gatherer forebears, that's a nearly forty-fold rise. We need to be sure that sugar is nothing more than a fatty "empty calorie" if we're going to see a rise like that.

As a prelude to our discussion of sugar, let's take a moment to define it. Glucose and fructose molecules make up table sugar, the white granulated material we buy in the enormous paper bags. The sugar content is split 50-50. A popular sweetener in food, high-fructose corn syrup (HFCS), is generally 55 percent fructose and 45 percent glucose. Table sugar and high fructose corn syrup are, thus, interchangeable terms. Table sugar and HFCS make up the majority of the 150 pounds of sugar consumed by the average American.

Table sugar and HFCS are both converted down into glucose and fructose when we eat them. After that, the process is the same as it was for the glucose derived from grains. When blood glucose levels rise, the pancreas releases insulin, which then transports the glucose to the body's tissues. Fat is deposited in the adipose tissue when the tissues are unable to absorb it. Again, fat accumulation isn't caused by consuming fat; rather, it's caused by consuming too much sugar.

When it comes to the metabolic consequences of fructose, they are considerably more harmful. fructose can only be broken down by certain cells in the human body, unlike glucose. Even though fructose is considered a poison by the body, its removal from the circulation is a primary goal. A little amount of fructose may be burnt for energy in the liver, as can other poisons. Fat molecules are formed from the remaining fatty acids, which are subsequently transported into the circulation as triglycerides (fat). Our blood triglyceride levels rise as a result of eating more sugar. Triglyceride levels in the circulation are a well-known indicator of cardiovascular disease risk. "

Fat deposits in the liver are another side effect of an overindulgent diet high in fructose, as is seen in alcoholics. As a result, "nonalcoholic fatty liver disease" is the term used to describe it. Fatty liver from fructose overconsumption may also lead to liver dysfunction and even liver failure, much as fatty liver from overconsumption of alcohol (Tappy 2012; Abdelmalek et al. 2010; Lim et al. 2010). Precursor to full-blown diabetes, insulin resistance, appears to be linked to fatty liver disease (Smith and Adams 2011; Stanhope and Havel 2008). Since sugar consumption has skyrocketed in recent decades, I don't think it's a coincidence that diabetes rates have skyrocketed at the same time

Fructose and AGEs are the two main culprits.

What happens when we consume more fructose than our liver can handle and fructose enters our blood stream? People produce advanced glycation products. Sugar molecules in the circulation (such glucose or fructose) bind to proteins on cells in our bodies and generate AGEs. AGEs can cause a variety of health problems (blood vessels, eyes, kidneys, brain, etc.). When a sugar molecule attaches to a cell, the cell's structure and function are compromised. Permanently. There will never be another cell like it. Since the body's inability to remove glucose from the bloodstream causes diabetes, AGEs accumulate throughout the patient's whole body. This is why diabetes has such a wide range of consequences (heart, blood vessels, brain, nerves, eyes, kidneys).

HOW TO CURE A MIGRAINE WITH FOOD

AGEs caused by glucose aren't as much of an issue for folks who don't have a problem eliminating glucose from the bloodstream.

But when it comes to protein with fructose, fructose is 10 times more likely than glucose to generate an AGE. Fructose in the blood would have to be much less concentrated to trigger AGE-mediated tissue damage. Non-diabetics are also at risk from AGEs, which have been linked to a variety of health problems (Yaffe and colleagues, 2011; Maillard-Lefebvre et al, 2009), with fructose once again implicated as the cause of this harm. Degenerative disorders of the brain, such as Alzheimer's and Parkinson's, have been linked to the presence of AGEs in pathological indicators (Münch et al. 1998; Srikanth et al. 2011).

Appetite and Fructose

Fructose isn't the only sugar that's terrible for you. When it comes to controlling one's hunger, fructose is a sneaky thief. The increased production of leptin in the body as a result of sugar consumption is considered to help curb hunger. You feel full because your brain senses that you've just eaten, and this is a natural and acceptable feedback mechanism. The ingestion of fructose, on the other hand, has been linked to a decrease in leptin levels. This implies that consuming meals high in fructose may make you feel more hungry despite the calories you've just consumed because of the actions of leptin in the brain.

Just when you think things couldn't get any worse, new data suggests that fructose may be linked to cancer (Liu and Heaney 2011). Hunter-gatherers that migrate to a contemporary diet, one that includes a significant increase in sugar consumption, see a huge increase in cancer incidence. When sugar intake rises, cancer rates tend to increase as well, especially in post-agricultural cultures.

Sugar and fructose appear to have a link to cancer because of their ability to promote insulin resistance, which is linked to cancer. To remove glucose from the circulation, the pancreas has to secrete progressively more insulin. In that it keeps blood glucose levels from rising too high, this is a positive thing. However, it can lead to "pancreatic burnout" and the establishment of diabetes in the long run. Cancer cells, on the other hand, rely on insulin as a source of energy (Boyd 2003). They grow quicker with more insulin. Obesity and diabetes are well-known risk factors for cancer, and it's possible that this is the case here.

So if insulin is a cancer fuel, then we should avoid the insulin resistance-related pathological rises in insulin levels. What can we do to prevent insulin resistance? The most common modern food source of fructose, sugar, may be

THE BOOK'S ABOUT 65

avoided. As Gary Taubes (2011) explains, two of the world's foremost cancer doctors confessed to being terrified of sugar in a recent New York Times Magazine piece.

The End of the Story: Sugar

The evidence on sugar is now complete, so let's have a look. Sugar, on the other hand, is really delectable. We can't stop eating it since it's so good, especially when it's dissolved in a colourful bubbly drink.

Sugar, on the other hand, is devoid of nutrition and is the ultimate empty calorie. Additionally, it's extremely caloric since it has a tendency for causing huge insulin spikes that send glucose into fat cells for storage. It also induces fat accumulation in the liver, leading to liver disease and insulin resistance due to the peculiar way it is processed. As a result, the alarming rise in obesity and diabetes in recent decades, as well as the tragic and unprecedented epidemic of obesity and diabetes in youngsters, may be attributable in large part to this factor. Sugar intake is also a major factor in the development of arterial plaques that contribute to heart attacks and strokes. In addition, it may have a direct impact on cancer growth.

Robert Lustig, a professor of paediatrics in the Division of Endocrinology at the University of California–San Francisco, referred to sugar as a "poison" in a 2009 lecture entitled "Sugar: The Bitter Truth." It's simple to see why.

Omega-6 Fatty Acids are a third suspect.

You're not alone if you haven't heard of our third suspect. But you may rest guaranteed that you've consumed considerably more of it than our pre-civilized predecessors ever did. What is an omega-6 fatty acid, and why do we need it?

It's essential that we first comprehend fat in order to grasp omega-6 (also known as "n-6") acids. With glucose and protein in the macronutrients, fat is one of them. Fats are essential to human health and survival, despite decades of misdirected attacks on the subject by the food industry. If you've ever heard somebody talk about fat as if it were a one-size-fits-all commodity, you're not alone.

Triglycerides, a large molecule with three fatty acids connected to a glycerol backbone, are found in our meals. The pancreas releases enzymes that break down triglycerides into their component fatty acids, which are then absorbed into the bloodstream. After being taken into the bloodstream, these fatty acids might be further metabolised. When we ingest fat, our bodies "see" it as fatty acids. Because these fatty acids have a certain structure and shape, this dictates how they interact with the body.

Saturated and unsaturated fatty acids are the two main types of fatty acids. When all of the carbon atoms in a fatty acid are linked to hydrogen atoms, it is said to be "saturated." This means that it is completely "saturated" by hydrogen. Because all of a molecule's attachment sites are filled once it reaches saturation, it is far less likely to react with objects in its immediate vicinity. As a result, saturated fatty acids are extremely resistant to oxidation, which is why they are long-lasting and difficult to breakdown. Instead, unsaturated fats include carbon atoms that aren't hydrogen-bonded, which increases their reactivity when they come into touch with other substances. We have both monounsaturated and polyunsaturated fatty acids in the class of unsaturated fats. The prefix "mono" refers to the fact that monounsaturated fats contain only one carbon atom that is unbound by hydrogen. As a result, they are less stable and more reactive than saturated fats, which are more stable and less reactive. They are the least stable and most reactive fatty acid species, polyunsaturated fats (also called PUFAs), have two or more carbon atoms that are not linked to hydrogen.

Our third suspect, omega-6 fatty acids, are the most reactive of the fatty acid species since they are a kind of PUFA. Fat is essential to our survival, unlike our first two suspicions, carbohydrates and sugar. As with fructose, the issue here is in how much we ingest.

Vegetable and seed oils, which have just recently entered the human diet as major sources of omega-6 fatty acids, are the primary sources in our modern diet. You can't just grab a handful of sunflower or soybean seeds and squeeze your way to a container of oil. The oils must be extracted from plants or seeds using chemical or mechanical methods that have just recently been established. For the pre-agricultural ancestors, omega-6 fatty acid intake was much lower than it is now since they didn't have the technology to extract these oils.

inflammation, eicosanoids, and the fatty acid linoleic acid

For more than just impressing your pals, the term "eicosanoids" refers to an entire family of signalling molecules that are crucial to our body's ability to respond to and respond to inflammation and our immune system. It is derived from the fatty acids in our cell membranes, and the fatty acid that is employed specifies the specific eicosanoid. Eicosanoids produced in the cell membrane by converting omega-6 fatty acids to omega-3 fatty acids do not cause inflammation. Because of this, the number of inflammatory chemicals produced by our bodies is directly influenced by our cells' ratio of omega-6 to omega-3 (also known as "n-3"). The more omega-6 fatty acids there are compared to omega-3 fatty acids in our cell membranes, the more inflammation there is in our body tissues as a whole.

Why is the ratio of omega-6 to omega-3 in our cell membranes so important? Our food choices. The ratio of omega-6 to omega-3 fatty acids in our pre-agricultural ancestors' diets is thought to have been 1:1 or 2:1. Nowadays, because of widespread usage of industrially manufactured oils, this ratio is believed to be between ten to twenty-five times. Inflammatory eicosanoids are then produced as a result of this incorrect ratio, which causes a lot of inflammation.

Irritation is a serious concern since inflammation plays an important role in many diseases—including most—if not all—illnesses. civilization's An abundance of data from epidemiological and animal research demonstrates a link between this misaligned ratio and the development of cardiovascular disease, autoimmune disease, a variety of cancers as well as mental health problems (Simopoulos 2002).

So, what are our options for regaining control of our swollen, swollen bodies? Omega-6: Omega-3 ratio should be 2:1, which is what our bodies are accustomed to. There are two possible approaches to this problem:

• Option 1: Increase the intake of n-3 fatty acids. If we consume too much n-6, we may adjust by eating more n-3, bringing the ratio back to its original state. Omega-3 fatty acids, which are abundant in fish oil, are often hailed by health authorities as a way to lower your risk of heart disease. Omega-3 fatty acids are still polyunsaturated, which is a drawback to this strategy. Because of their great reactivity, polyunsaturated fatty acids are the most prevalent fatty acid subtype, as we learned in our lesson on fatty acids. As a result, free radicals can be generated within the body, causing tissue damage. This oxidation (basically an oxygen reaction, similar to the one that causes an apple to brown when exposed to air) is particularly dangerous. However, if nothing is done, we're only making a choice between bad options.

• Option 2: Reducing our diet of omega-6 fatty acids is a more logical way to restore the omega-6 to omega-3 ratio. By maintaining a low level of oxidising reactive PUFAs, this procedure not only restores the ratio to its natural state.

Some Thoughts on the Use of Trans Fats

HOW TO CURE A MIGRAINE WITH FOOD

Animal fats were outlawed in fast food restaurants in the mid-1980s, which turned out to be one of the most disastrous public health mistakes in recent memory. Unsubstantiated claims that lard used to cook French fries and other foods was a dietary evil were the basis for this as well.

As a result, partly hydrogenated vegetable oils, such as Crisco and margarine, began to replace animal fat in commercial kitchens across the country. Vegetable oils that have been partly hydrogenated are those that have been chemically changed to behave more like animal fats. Oils that are normally liquid at room temperature are solidified with this process, making them more stable and improving their cooking qualities in the process. As a result of the chemical process, partly hydrogenated oils are also trans fat. As a result of hydrogenation, trans fat is an unsaturated fat with a distinctive three-dimensional structure. Because trans fats were not a part of our diet until the last century, it's not unexpected that their unusual structure causes all kinds of mayhem when they're integrated into our cell membranes. Some studies have shown that trans fats are associated to a wide range of health problems including heart disease (Mozaffarian et al. 2006; Chajès et al. 2008; Stender and Dyerberg 2004). Fortunately, even the mainstream health community has realised the hazards of partly hydrogenated oils, which were long considered a "healthy alternative" to animal fat. For the first time, common sense has won in the popular dietary arena.

Your best bet is to stick with what you know.

Returning to the Plan

Almost as ingrained in our cultural consciousness as the idea that whole grains are an essential component of a nutritious diet is the assumption that animal fat clogs the arteries and that vegetable fats assist keep them clear. Mainstream medical experts have been reiterating this message for years now. Animal fat was once thought to be unhealthy for the arteries, thus the American Heart Association advised those with heart problems to use vegetable fat instead. This advice has been around for decades. And it's a stance that's held for over half a century despite a growing body of facts refuting it and receiving no substantial scientific backing (Siri-Tariano et al. 2010). It is the cornerstone upon which the vast majority of conventional dietary advice is based.

As it turns out, there is a growing body of data indicating the contrary. The use of vegetable fat in place of animal fat does not only provide little protection against heart disease, but rather makes it worse. In a research published in February 2013 in the British Medical Journal, this was made clear (Ramsden

THE BOOK'S ABOUT 69

et al.). Even more unfortunate, the data was really collected forty years ago. It turned out that the study's "missing" data from the Sydney Diet Heart Study was really the basis for the paper's reanalysis. Between 1966 and 1973, researchers studied 458 males between the ages of thirty-nine and fifty-nine who had just experienced a heart attack. Saturated fat was replaced with vegetable fat in the diets of half of the men who participated in the study. As a result, they used safflower oil, which is a particularly potent source of omega-6. The other half of the study, known as the "control group," was not instructed to alter their diet in any way. The findings were shocking to everyone who believed that animal fat was hazardous for the heart. According to this study, people who ate a diet high in vegetable fats were 35 percent more likely to die of a heart attack and 29 percent more likely to die of any cause. Furthermore, despite having cholesterol levels nearly 20 points lower than those in the control group, they achieved this outcome.

To prevent artery hardening, which in turn increases our risk of heart attacks and other ailments, we've been instructed to consume more vegetable fat rather than animal fat. It turns out that this counsel is not only contradictory to evolution, but it is also completely backward.

But even though I'm convinced it will eventually fade out, the assumption that animal fat causes heart disease still persists. It's a belief that hasn't been based on thorough scientific research, but rather on a combination of arrogance, shoddy science, and rushed public policy (Taubes 2008). Good science will win out in the end, and the theory will crumble under its own weight. For the first time in the history of mainstream nutrition, a positive transformation will take place.

The Final Word on Omega-6 Fatty Acids

There aren't large enough levels of linoleic acids in the typical American diet to be harmful, but the quantity we consume causes our bodies to become more prone to inflammation, which is a contributing factor to the development of nearly all modern illnesses. Animal fat is better for you than veggie fat, contrary to common opinion. And trans fats should be kept in the lab, not in your kitchen. "

Dairy is suspect number four.

Our ancestors started keeping animals for their milk as soon as agriculture and animal husbandry were developed. Milk is one of the best sources of full nourishment. However, humans haven't drunk other animals' milk for the most

HOW TO CURE A MIGRAINE WITH FOOD

of their time on our planet. As a result, milk, or dairy in general, should be considered a potential health hazard in our modern diet.

There are several advantages to drinking milk. While cereal grains have adapted to keep people from eating them through the natural selection process, milk is designed solely for consumption by animals. It is intended to be a mammal's only source of food and energy throughout its formative years. It includes all nine necessary amino acids, is rich in vitamins and minerals, and provides a well-balanced combination of carbohydrate, protein, and fat. Milk, in many respects, is the ideal nourishment for a baby. Human milk is a kind of it that has been consumed by humans for as long as we have been on this planet. Milk has been a part of our diet for a long time, and our genome has had time to adjust. Only the eating of non-human milk is a very new occurrence... Nonhuman milk consumption has thus far been found to have no significant relation to the illnesses of civilization. This is likely due to the fact that nonhuman milk is so similar to our own. However, despite the fact that milk does not appear to have the disease-causing potential of the other candidates we've explored, it can cause some issues for certain people.

Lactose and Milk Intolerance

Lactose, a molecule made up of one molecule of glucose and one molecule of galactose, is the primary source of sugar in milk. Lactase breaks down lactose into glucose and galactose before it can be absorbed. We get bloated, gassy, and other unpleasant symptoms if it isn't broken down before entering our digestive system. During infancy and early childhood, all people produce an abundance of lactase because our bodies anticipate to be fueled by our mothers' milk. Lactase production declines with age for the majority of us, albeit the extent of this decline varies widely by ethnicity. Lactase production is lowest in people of African and Asian heritage, whereas those of Northern European ancestry may never decrease at all. If you've got lactose intolerance, you'll feel awful after eating dairy products because of how much lactose they contain. Lactose sensitivity can be alleviated by fermented dairy products such as yoghurt and cheese, which have very low lactose content.

A sensitivity to lactose in milk

Milk contains a protein type known as casein. Species-specific casein can be discovered in cows, but it isn't the same casein found in humans. This change in casein protein composition can cause an allergic response in a limited proportion of persons. Wheezing, hives, and vomiting are all possible side effects. In young children, it is most frequent, but many grow out of it.

If casein is not entirely broken down prior to its absorption into the circulation, it may pose a risk. A healthy digestive tract breaks down casein into its individual amino acids before it enters the bloodstream. As a result of our leaky gut, casein can enter the bloodstream unchecked, which can lead to a variety of health issues. Systemic inflammation and an increased risk of autoimmune disease are two possible outcomes if it enters the bloodstream. Casein, on the other hand, offers a few advantages over gluten.

Nonhuman milk's casein, while not identical to human casein, is nonetheless closely connected to it because it is a protein produced by other animals. Gluten, on the other hand, is a plant protein that does not resemble anything human systems produce. As a result, if gluten enters the bloodstream, it is far more likely to be identified as an alien substance. A leaky gut must also be present for milk casein to enter the bloodstream in the first place. In the past, we've spoken about how ingesting plant lectins, such as those present in wheat, can lead to leaky stomachs. There is no way to get casein protein into the bloodstream when we're avoiding foods that cause a leaky gut in the first place. Casein is no longer a concern if the lining of the digestive tract remains intact.

Dairy intake has been linked to an increased risk of cancer, according to some. A small number of epidemiological studies have indicated that people with cancer were more likely to have ingested dairy than those who were not in those communities (Fairfield et al. 2004; Larsson, Bergkuist, and Wolk 2004). Other population studies, on the other hand (Moorman and Terry 2004), have not established a relationship between high-fat dairy intake and cancer (and vice versa) (Cho et al. 2004; Larsson, Bergkuist, and Wolk 2005). According to research (Miller et al. 2003; O'Shea et al. 2000), conjugated linoleic acid, a component of dairy fat, inhibits the development of cancer cells in tissue culture, which might explain this conclusion. Eating dairy, as long as the fat has not been eliminated (i.e., no low- or nonfat products), may lessen your risk of some types of cancer, according to these research.

The Bottom Line on Dairy

Except for those who are lactose intolerant or allergic to casein, there are no compelling reasons to avoid dairy, especially if you've eliminated the other components of your diet that harm your digestive tract's walls. Just steer clear of the low-fat and no-fat options, which are essentially just sugar and protein from milk, stripped of any of the beneficial fats that may help prevent cancer.

The Ending Conclusion

HOW TO CURE A MIGRAINE WITH FOOD

These three dietary ingredients, sugar, gluten grains, and omega-6 fatty acids, have an obvious and extremely reasonable relationship with modern civilization's ailments. Before agriculture, none of them were significant components of the human diet, and each has biological processes well proven by which it leads to civilization's diseases:

Trying to comprehend the entire burden of these diseases today is practically difficult. Our hospitals and clinics are overcrowded, putting an enormous strain on our health care system, and inflicting incalculable agony and suffering as a result of these very things. Furthermore, the fact that the vast majority of these tragedies may be avoided is both worrisome and heartening. Eventually, if everyone changed their diets in accordance with the present rules, I would be out of a job (and no, the health care business is not conspiring to keep a continual supply of consumers).

It goes without saying that this new perspective on a healthy diet compelled me to alter my own eating habits—and to do it in a way that was at odds with everything I'd previously been taught. My migraines disappeared as a direct result, but there were many other pleasant side benefits as well. As it turns out, I'm not the only one who has had this happen. I started hearing accounts from other migraineurs who had made similar changes to their diets when I understood how effective it was for me. Many long-term migraine sufferers, like me, were ecstatic at the end of their suffering.

Another affliction of modern civilization is migraine.

I can't help but believe that migraine, like so many other diseases, is a sickness of civilization based on my own and other people's personal experiences with it. This isn't a surprise in retrospect. We didn't become Earth's most populous species over the last 2.5 million years by being forced to puke in a dark cave every other day. Migraines must now be added to the ever-expanding list of human ailments. The fact that headaches may be avoided totally by changing our food and way of life is a testament to the notion that migraines aren't only a curse for some people. In addition, we now have a clear road to freedom from migraines thanks to this new understanding of migraine.

A New Look at the Migraine Epidemic

We learned in Chapter 2 that when our own migraine risk level rises over a certain threshold, our brains can activate the migraine process. Before I began eating an ancient diet, I frequently crossed the line. Even on a migraine-free day, I was never far from the threshold because of a strong family history of

THE BOOK'S ABOUT 73

migraines (unfavourable genetics) and the unpredictable sleep schedule that comes with taking regular hospital calls.. Figure 3a depicts my own migraine risk level based on the methodology described in chapter 2 of this book.

Figure 3a: Before I started eating an ancestral diet, my migraines looked like this on a daily basis. My migraine risk level was never far from the threshold because of a strong family history and an unpredictable sleep cycle, despite the benefit of a magnesium supplement.

Just about anything might send me over the edge, as you can see. For example, a bad night's sleep, skipping lunch, or an afternoon cup of caffeinated coffee would quickly send me into the throbbing-skull zone depicted in figure 3b.

The caffeine in a cup of coffee was all it took to raise my migraine risk beyond the threshold before making the move to an ancestral diet (Figure 3b).

When I first started having migraines, I was certain that I was doing everything I could to prevent them. I even accepted that they may strike at any time, and I felt I was doing everything I could to prevent them.

Things have drastically changed since then. As a result of following an ancestral diet, I'm able to maintain my migraine risk far lower than I ever expected to be (figure 3c).

Figure 3c shows that my migraine risk level has decreased significantly after I began following an ancestral diet.

When it comes to properly comprehending just how far away the threshold is, we need to shift our mindset (figure 3d).

At this point in my ancestral diet, I'm so far from the threshold that I have to shift my viewpoint just to see it!

Everything that formerly would have sent me over the edge no longer does so since my baseline risk is so low. When I'm drinking coffee in a café, I can sit next to an olfactorily challenged man wearing overpowering fragrance and munching on nuts and blue cheese without feeling any discomfort in my brain because of the weight of an ancient diet (figure 3e).

Figure 3e: My migraine risk is so low thanks to an ancestral diet that even the combination of several of my old foes isn't enough to push me over the edge.

HOW TO CURE A MIGRAINE WITH FOOD

Our greatest weapon against migraine has been forgotten for all these years—far better than any drug or supplement. Absolutely nothing beats an ancestral diet when it comes to reducing our migraine risk.

What Gave Us Them To Miss It?

The fact that we've overlooked something so obvious for so long is astounding when you stop to consider it. As we all know, food may cause migraines, and many sufferers try to pinpoint exactly what they consume that causes their attacks. Sugar, wheat, and vegetable and seed oils aren't likely to appear on any list of dietary migraine causes. Surely this isn't true. Because these foods are so helpful in preventing migraines, why didn't we learn about them sooner?

These substances are so common in our diets that we haven't recognised their role in migraines (and other illnesses of civilization, for that matter) for a long time. Consider the situation of lung cancer for a moment. Cigarette smoking is widely recognised as the leading cause of lung cancer in the modern world. We know this because the risk of lung cancer in smokers is ten to twenty times greater than in nonsmokers. As a result, the link between smoking and lung cancer has been quite straightforward to establish.

If everyone smoked, what would happen? When investigating the origins of an illness, it is common to begin by comparing the dietary, lifestyle, and genetic profiles of persons with and those without the condition. Smoking causes lung cancer, but if everyone smoked, we'd have no way of knowing. Even while not everyone who smokes will develop cancer, there will be people with lung cancer and those without it, and the smoking rates in these two groups will be same. This time, we'll focus on what separates each group. While genetic abnormalities or exposure to chemicals such as arsenic may be considered the most significant risk factors, we may be forgetting the underlying reason.

Wheat, sugar, and plant oils, the contemporary diet's disease-causing components, are the same. Because of the agricultural revolution, they've become a mainstay in almost every modern society. Migraine may not have been discovered if it hadn't been for the isolated communities of humans who were never influenced by the agricultural revolution.

The only thing that's left to explain is how the current diet causes migraines. Migraines haven't been discussed as a major cause of death and disease in our society, but wheat, sugar, and omega-6 fats have. It's not clear why these dietary culprits are responsible for migraines.